The Adventure Continues

The Adventure Continues

Living with Amyotrophic Lateral Sclerosis (ALS)

By

Marcel LaPerriere

Published by Marcel LaPerriere, 2019
Printed in the United States of America
Distributed by Ingram Spark
ISBN: 978-0-578-52488-7

Book design by Dana G. Anderson

The events and experiences that follow are all true, based on the author's
recollection of them. In some situations, names, identities, and other
specifics of individuals have been changed in order to protect their privacy.

Dedication

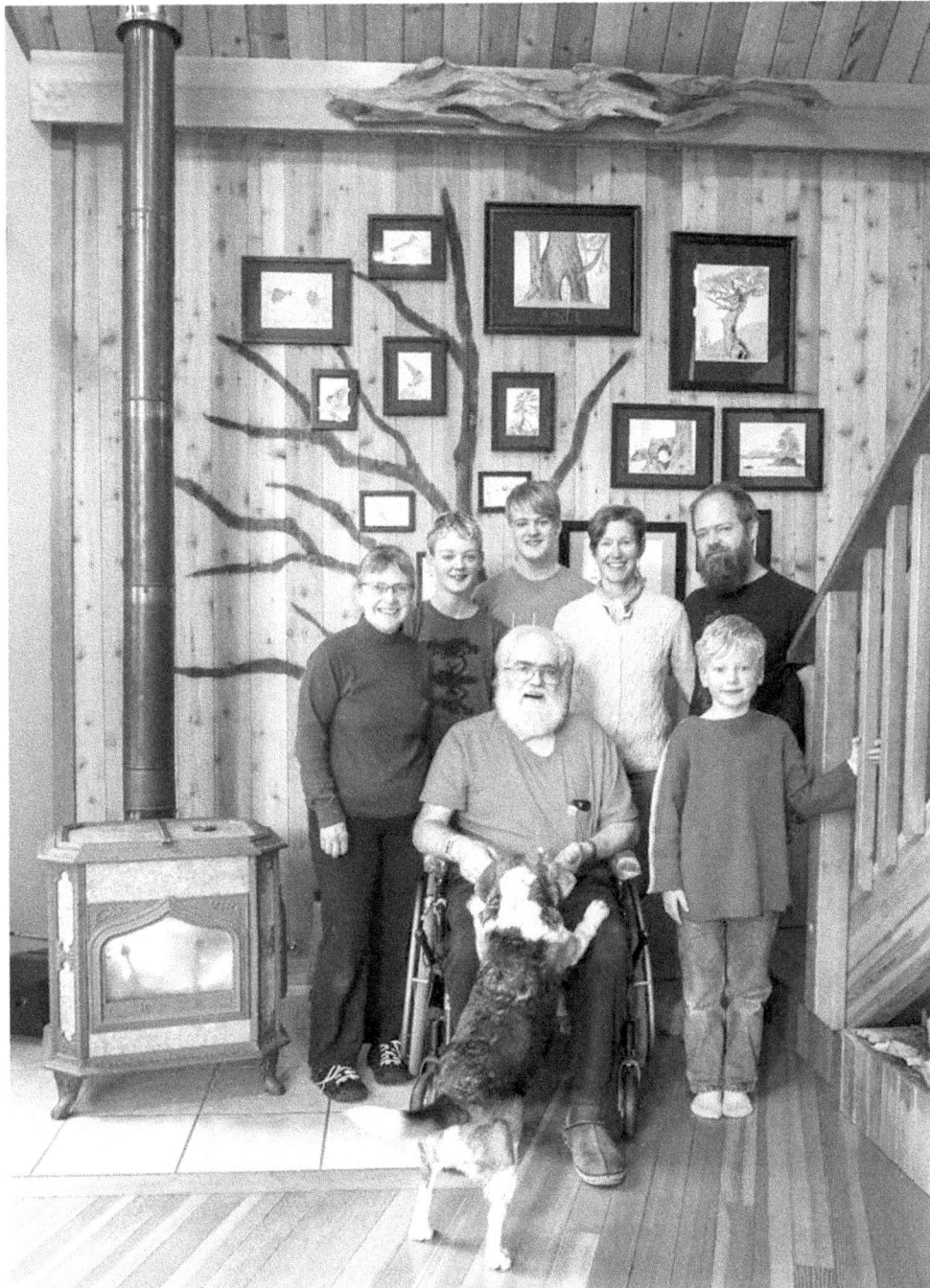

To my Family.

Back row: Connie, Nate 13, Blake 17, Jenn and Zach
Front row: Me and Dane, aka Lucky 8.
And of course, Bella. We tried and tried to get her to face the camera.

Table of Contents

Foreword

"You have fast progression ALS," was what I heard on February 2, 2019. As many of you know, these very words changed my life. As I struggled to understand what this meant, and how I was going to deal with it, I started looking for stories of other people who were dealing with having ALS. Someone had posted a link to Marcel LaPerriere's book, *Just Another Adventure: Living with Amyotrophic Lateral Sclerosis*. I downloaded and read it. I'm so glad I did. Marcel really explains what his experience with ALS has been like. What really struck me was the underlying message of hope and life. "Live your life" was his message, not "live to die." I have to remind myself of that every day. Even the hard days when I discover I can no longer do something that I have done up to that point. His book made me laugh and cry. So, I left a review. Turns out Marcel is on the same ALS Facebook page that I had recently joined, and we found each other. He asked if I would be interested in writing the Foreword, and would I include my experience with ALS. Never having done this before, and totally out of my comfort zone, I said "Yes." My hope is that my experience will help someone else, like Marcel's first book, helped me.

Marcel's book really hit me because I believe in positive thinking and could see that throughout his book. However, I am prone to negative thinking. I really have to work hard to stay in a positive zone most of the time. Then I was diagnosed with ALS. Reading his book reminded me I have a family to live for. There are milestones for my kids that I want to be there for. I may not be, but I try not to spend too much time on that. My kids are 18,16 and 12 years of age as I write this. I want to be there for them as long as I can. Marcel reminds us that even as we can do less, there are still plenty of things to live for. We just have to figure out what that is for each of us. His essays were a breath of fresh air for me. They reinforced the feelings I knew would help me navigate this disease. Many of his essays were funny. He poked fun at himself. I've been able to do that a few times, and it is so much better than crying.

Somewhere around Spring 2017 I began having trouble lifting my left foot properly and started tripping. I fell quite a few times. Around December 2017 I went in to see my doctor. I was referred to a neurologist who ordered a foot brace (no more tripping over my own foot). He also ordered an EMG, MRI, and X-ray. We were trying to find out what was causing my drop foot. A slipping vertebra was thought to be the culprit. October 4, 2018, I had anterior spinal fusion surgery. In December 2018, my family started commenting on my speech, which sounded like I'd had a stroke or was drunk or had a thick tongue. I was also noticing muscle twitches. Again, I went back to my doctor, who referred me to the same neurologist who gave me a blood test. The results came back negative, for what I don't remember, but he then sent me to the specialist in neuromuscular diseases. I saw her in January 2019, when she looked at the twitches in my arm. I then had an EMG and an MRI. She told me on February 2, 2019, that I had ALS. It took me about a week to start looking into ALS. During that first week, in the middle of the night, I had two separate panic attacks. At the first one, my husband, Brian, was still up. I got up and talked to him, which helped immensely.

However, the second time, everyone else in the house was asleep, and I had to talk myself out of the anxiety I was feeling. I started thinking about the positive things in my life, and somehow talked myself out of the panicky feeling I was having. I was eventually able to go to sleep. I realized that this was going to keep happening unless I started talking about it. I talked to anyone who would listen. Family, friends, co-workers, anybody. Talking really helped. And then I found Marcel's book.

This book will be like the first one. My hope is that it reaches many more people who have ALS or know someone with ALS. As Marcel points out, we all have something to live for. We just have to find out what that is.

Susan Emerson
California
May 2019

Introduction

At the summit of Mt. Slesse in the summer of 1974, my climbing partner, Greg, and I shook hands while admiring the 360-degree view. After looking back over the Northwest Ridge we had just climbed, I looked south across the Canadian border into Washington State, and then directly west. Though the distance is close to one hundred miles, under those perfectly clear blue skies, I could see past the city of Vancouver to the Straits of Georgia. I could even see what looked like little toys but were, in fact, a couple of British Columbia ferries motoring to and from Vancouver Island. As I was overcome by the endless beauty that lay before me, my only regret was not sharing the moment with my wife, Connie, and our infant son, Zach. I didn't know it at the time, but seeing the ocean off in the distance put into motion a daydream that would change the trajectory of our lives.

Sadly, one of the worst airplane crashes to that date occurred on Mt. Slesse when a Canadair North Star four-engine aircraft slammed into the mountain near the summit on December 9, 1956, killing 62 people. As Greg on I sat on the summit, we talked about some of the crash debris still defying

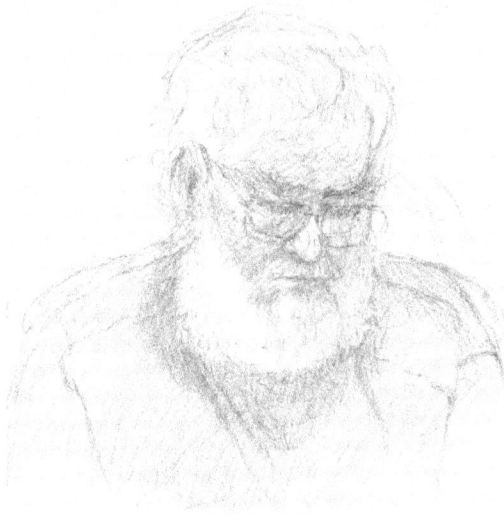

gravity as it clung to the near-vertical rock. We talked about how death can come swiftly and without warning like it had for the people in the plane on that fateful day in December eighteen years before. We also talked about the risk of climbing and how a couple of climbers we knew had recently fallen to their deaths while climbing on the Eiger. Of course, being young, we felt invincible. But as we descended the mountain, we came across some of the luggage, clothing and other debris from the crash, and for some reason that affected me much more than seeing the metal parts of the plane. The luggage and clothing were a physical reminder that many people had been killed on the very mountain we were now climbing down. Seeing the clothing was a personification that made me more empathetic to the victims of the crash. Once again it made me realize how fragile life can be, and that made me find an adventurous sport that I could share with my family. That realization brought me back to my daydream.

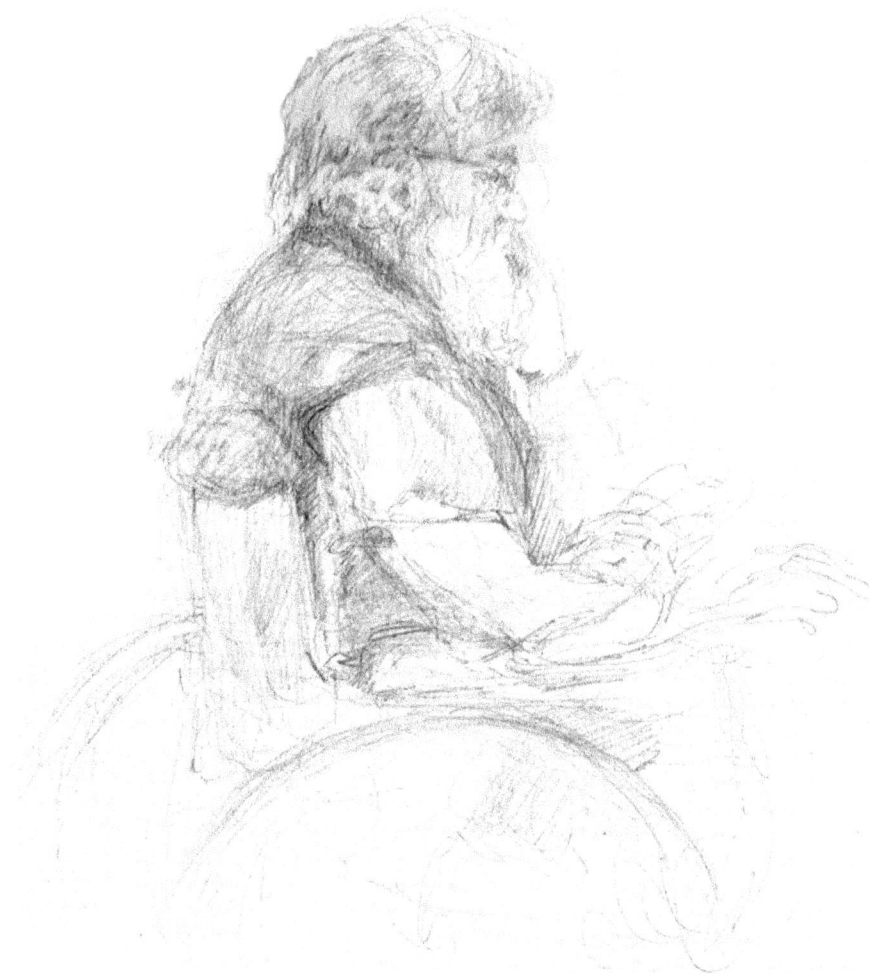

After a climb, I was always anxious to get home to tell Connie about the adventure. This time, I was much more anxious to tell her that I had dreamed up a plan that would allow us to share our adventures together. After giving Connie a quick rundown of the climbing, I told her about my daydream. I told her, as I stood on the summit of Mt. Slesse, that I saw sailboats sailing on the waters of the inland passage and out the Straits of Juan de Fuca. With the distance from the mountain top to the ocean, I couldn't actually have seen boats sailing, yet in my mind I did. I went on to tell Connie if we learned to sail and owned a sailboat, instead of me going off climbing and leaving her home with a baby, as a family we could enjoy an adventure each weekend.

Growing up in Colorado, the only boats I'd ever been on were the rental pedal boats in the Denver City Park lake, and I'm not sure that Connie had ever been on a boat. Yet, as young and crazy as we were, Connie agreed that it sounded fun. Maybe the seed had been planted a few years earlier when as a school girl, Connie had read Robin Lee Graham's book *Dove*, about his adventure as a teenager sailing around the world solo. At the time I had not read that book or any book about sailing, so I have no idea what sparked my daydream. Whatever the spark was, I'm darn glad it lit the fire in both of us to spend most of our adult lives living on or near the water.

Within a few weeks of climbing Mt. Slesse, we had both read a dozen books about sailing adventures, or books on how to sail, and we bought our first sailboat; a little eight-foot-long fiberglass dingy. Soon the little boat was in the water, and I was teaching myself how to sail. And when I wasn't sailing, I was taking care of Zach, while Connie was teaching herself to sail. Only when we felt confident of our abilities, did we all three climb into the little sailboat, and only when there was not much wind. We sure weren't going to endanger our baby by being overly anxious to get on the water.

Not only was my daydream our inspiration for learning to sail, but it was the genesis of us living on three different sailboats for an accumulated twenty-five years. Also, a line could be drawn from our love of boating and oceans to the pathway that ultimately led us to Alaska and all the adventure we've had living here. Plus, our love of life on and near the water is now being passed onto our three grandsons through our son. And, that makes both of us happy.

My daydream taught me more than anything to live life to the fullest and to live that life with the ones you love. Experience has also taught me that things don't always go as planned. I sure didn't plan on getting amyotrophic lateral sclerosis (ALS). Not even in my worst nightmares did I ever envision being confined to a wheelchair and not being able to talk. But that doesn't mean I'm bitter. Even with ALS, I'm blessed in too many ways to count. I take comfort that I still am married to that same amazing woman who agreed with me all those years ago that we should learn to sail. That same woman who, despite the bumps of life, is still putting up with me. The same woman I frequently see playing with our grandsons as if she was their age and not of Medicare age. The same woman I'm always happy to see when I wake up in the morning and who makes my life such a joy.

You, too, can find happiness even if you or a loved one is dealing with ALS. It's not easy, and for sure, you must work at it. But happiness is so much better than all the negative things that one can dwell on when living with a disease like ALS. Life isn't always fair, and both life and love can be fragile. Further, I've cheated death more than once. I feel lucky to be able to say that, which makes life even more valuable for me.

In this book, I hope to share with you more adventures and how I deal with a disease that I know is killing me. I'm trying to look at ALS as just another adventure, and I'm happy that five years into the journey of living with ALS, the adventure continues.

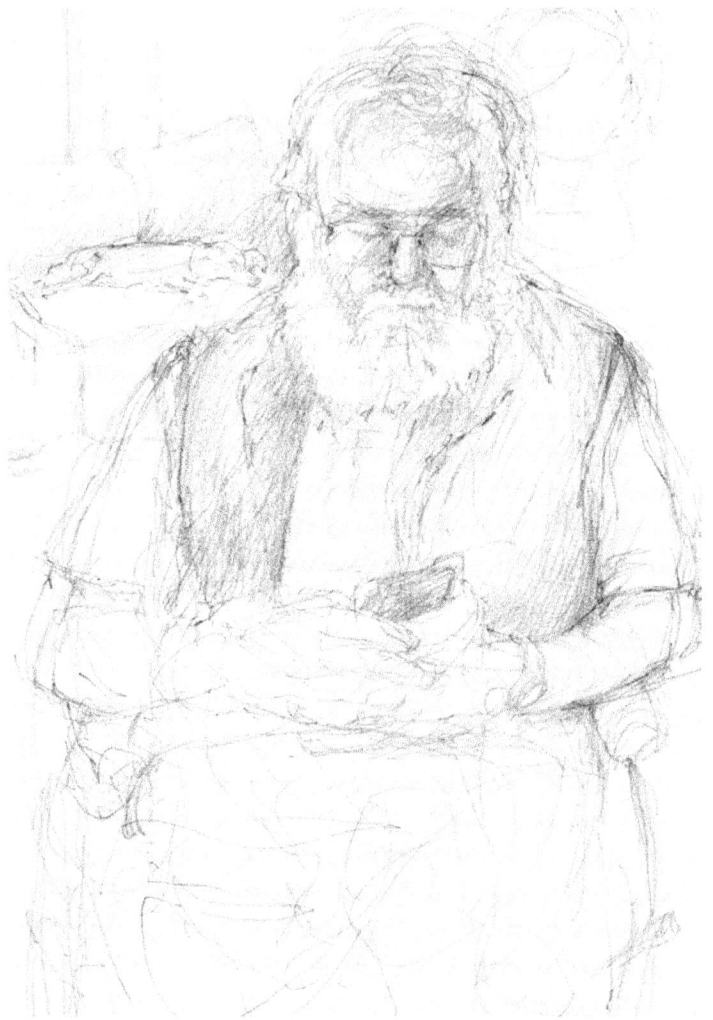

Sketches of Marcel are by his cousin, Michelle LaPerriere, in July of 2018.

Timeline

Approximate Date	Approximate Age	Symptoms
January 2014	61	Started noticing that my voice would sort of slur or break in the evenings.
August 2014	61 1/2	Connie noticed for the first time that I was slurring my voice.
October 2014	61 3/4	After visiting with our family doctor we were sent to see a neurologist at Virginia Mason. I started confusing words when I talked -- simple things like saying bird when I wanted to say seagull.
November 2014	61 3/4	Neurologist suggested that I possibly had primary progressive aphasia. Meanwhile I continued to loose my voice. I entered what I call the drunk phase, because I sounded drunk when I talked.
February 2015	62	Neurologist said that she was fairly sure I had primary progressive aphasia.
March 2015	62	Neurologist suggested that I might have spasmodic dysphonia.
April 2015	62	Neurologist Dr. Elliot suggested that I be tested for acromegaly.
June 2015	62 1/2	Acromegaly was confirmed.

July 2015	62 1/2	Met with an endocrinologist, because my tongue was growing. She put me on a three times day injection of a drug called Octreotide.
August 2015	62 1/2	Started the Octreotide injections and they made me very sick. I was sick for the whole month and my voice got weaker and weaker. The tongue started to shrink.
September 2015	62 1/2	Had an infusion of Sandostatin Depot. That, too, made me sick. The tongue continued to shrink back to normal size. My voice continued to fade away.
October 2015	62 3/4	Had surgery to remove the tumor on my pituitary gland.
October 2015	62 3/4	Bad reaction to penicillin caused ethermal multiforme. I ended up in the hospital for a week -- four days in critical care.
January 2016	63	Balance was getting bad.
January 2016	63	Voice -- totally gone.
February 2016	63	Dr. Elliott suggested that I might have pseudo-bulbar palsy.
February 2016	63	Walking okay but breathing is becoming more and more labored.
July 2017	64 1/2	Balance issues are found to be from a disorder called semicircular canal dehiscence.
Summer 2017	64	Walking became harder and harder. Started using a walker off and on.
Fall 2017	64 3/4	Started having problems with constipation.
February 2018	65	Attended an ALS Clinic. My ankles were very swollen. Ended up in the ER at Virginia Mason and two nights in the hospital.
March 2018	65	Had a PEG feeding tube installed.
March 2018	65	Walking declined to the point that I ended up in a wheelchair.
April 2018	65 1/4	Start process to get an electric wheelchair
April 2018	65 1/4	Bedsores start becoming an issue.
May 2018	65 1/4	A mysterious bedsore with broken skin forms right behind my right big toe.

June 2018	65 1/2	Measured for a power wheelchair on the 13th of June.
June 2018	65 1/2	June 18th purchased a newly converted, slightly used 2017 handicap van. Delivered in Aug. 2018
June 2018	65 1/2	Get new electric wheelchair
July 2018	65 1/2	Losing more and more dexterity in my fingers – especially on the left hand.
October 2018	65 3/4	Having troubles with my eyelids not opening up as they should.
November 2019	65 3/4	Breathing is getting hard and harder. Start the process to get an noninvasive ventilator called a Trilogy Ventilator.
Feb-19	66	Lots of fasciculations at night, mostly on my left side's, elbow, kneecap and calf, and my left hand's thumb, index finger and middle finger.
February 2019	66	Swallowing is getting harder. Even ice cream or applesauce is hard to swallow.
March 2019	66	When I sleep on my right side in the fetal position, then try to straighten my right leg, I can't and need to use my arms to push the leg straight.
April 2019	66 1/4	My neck is getting weak and is often sore. I have a hard time nodding, "Yes," but still can shake it, "No."
May 2019	66 1/4	Received my Trilogy machine as breathing continues to get harder.

Essays

The Dumb Things People Say and Do

29 June 2018

From time to time we all say or do dumb things. I sure have.

Now that I'm handicapped I've experienced a whole new level of dumb things that people say and do. As Alaskans, and people who used to own a gift shop, Connie and I have heard some doozies.

When we owned a store in Ketchikan, the big question that many tourists ask shortly after they come off the cruise ship is, "What is the elevation here?" The answer should be self-evident, since they stepped off an ocean-going cruise ship. Surprisingly, that question gets asked so frequently it has become a routine question to answer for anyone who works around tourists. The next most frequently asked question was, "Do you take American money?" Or, "will my American credit cards work here?" I was even asked once why there was an American flag flying from the building across the street from our store. I hope they got it when I answered, "Because that's the local Federal Building." A favorite was when a well-dressed man in his 50's asked me slowly in a loud voice, "DO…. YOU… SPEAK… ENGLISH?" If I had been thinking faster, instead of answering, "Yes," I should have mumbled some gibberish and then laughed. My all-time favorite dumb question by a tourist was when a woman asked a tour bus driver in Juneau, "Did they put the glacier so far from downtown so they could charge more for the tour?" I've also been asked where the best place is to see polar bears and even penguins –– penguins don't even live in Alaska or the Arctic.

Now there are new dumb things I'm hearing from my wheelchair. A man who works in my primary care doctor's office must assume that I'm deaf as well as mute. Whenever he sees me he always greets me in an extra loud voice. He doesn't do this with others and he must not have observed Connie or others talking to me in a normal voice. Several people slow their speaking when they talk to me. But what takes the cake is what happened to me last night. I was waiting in line for the doors to open for a Sitka Summer Music Festival concert, talking with a very nice lady whom I've known casually for several years. She'd ask me a few questions, and then I'd type my answer into the phone so that she could read it. Along with the questions, she was telling me all sorts of interesting ways I could get over ALS. As much as I wanted to, I didn't tell her that there are no cures for ALS. A few minutes after that conversation she grabbed a couple of programs for the night's music. She asked me if I wanted one, and when I shook my head "No," She then asked me, "Can you read?" Keep in mind that was after I'd typed into my phone a few things for her to read. I'm guessing that she equates the fact that I can't talk with a possible stroke, not knowing that a common symptom of ALS is losing one's ability to talk. She obviously hadn't thought it through. If I can write, I should be able to read.

We all do and say some dumb things. Maybe I'm lucky that I can't talk? It sure keeps me from joining my fellow humans by saying dumb things.

The Moth

2 July 2018

I have a confession to make. In today's world of the Internet a lot of people binge watch their favorite TV or Netflix series, like Orange is the New Black, or some other addicting show. I'm not watching all seven Harry Potter movies, or even The Lord of the Ring movies. My confession is the I've been binge listening to the podcast "The Moth."

"The Moth" is a series of human-interest stories told in front of live audiences around the world. A story told by a woman in Dublin, Ireland tells what it's like to be discriminated against because she is 3' 10." She tells how she teaches her 6th grade students to understand that people are different and not weirdos. A man within the walls of one of America's prisons tells about what it's like to be serving a life sentence for murder. And a former Vogue Magazine editor shares what it was like to live in a haunted apartment in Paris, France.

Here is another confession. As a guy who was raised Catholic, I think today, being Sunday, is a good day to bare my soul.

So, here goes. I'd love to present in the next Story Slam telling the people in that audience what it's like to not be able to speak. I'd be nervous, but I'd soon get over that, and get on with my story. Because ALS stole my ability to talk, I can never tell any audience what it's like to not be able to speak.

The Adventure Continues

I can't tell my story because I can't talk. The only way I could ever tell you, or anyone, what it's like not being able to talk is in writing.

Further Decline

9 July 2018

The one given with ALS is that there will always be more and more declining of body functions. As expected, this true for me, too.

Standing is getting harder and harder. I feel lucky that I can even stand. Four years into the journey of living with ALS, most people won't be standing at all. As much as I hate spending most of my day sitting in a wheel-chair, it could be much worse. I can still stand to wash a dish in the sink or grab something from a higher shelf.

Eating and drinking. Ugh. This is what I hate to admit. My ability to eat and drink by mouth is also evaporating away. Blended or soft foods are now almost a must. I can still enjoy some food by mouth, but most of my favorite foods are now things of the past. I'm definitely not looking forward to when all my nourishments must come to me by the PEG feeding tube. Drinking thin liquids is also getting increasingly harder and harder. Each morning I still make a cup of coffee, but it's a rare day when I can get the whole cup down. When I do finish off the cup, most of the coffee has dribbled down my chin, not got down my throat. I still sip on water all day long, but it's much the same for the water. My sips of water are down to about a half-teaspoon each, and much of that also doesn't go down where it should -- so, most of my liquids come from applesauce or hot cereal or go into the PEG.

The scariest decline that I'm facing now is the lack of coordination of my fingers. Simple things like putting a lid back on a jar are getting hard -- even something as simple as hitting my open mouth with a toothbrush. It shocked me when I hit my lower lip with the toothbrush instead of my open mouth. I had to put new toothpaste on the brush and start over. And, I'm having a harder and harder time typing -- both on the computer and on my phone. That scares the dickens out of me because my primary way of communicating is by typing.

Last week we had a week of very nice sunny weather, so I spent much of the day out on the deck sitting in the sun and listening to podcasts. I over used my legs by pulling or pushing myself around in the wheelchair, up and down ramps to the point that I had swelling and associated pain in all my joints from the hips down. This gave me an insight into what is coming. The pain made it hard for me to get in and out of bed, off and on the toilet, in and out of the shower, and dressing myself. I'm doing much better now, but that experience was an eye-opener. If we are going to do one more road trip, we have to do it before I need to rely on help for the things I've mentioned above.

As I was finishing writing this, I had a computer message from a young woman and mother that I follow on the British MND Facebook site. She was responding to a comment that I'd made on her earlier posting. She had posted that after a six-month period of depression, she had decided that she wasn't going to let MND/ALS define her. I had complimented her on that decision and her response was, "I learned that from you and Chris." (Chris is a man in Britain who is also keeping positive about his MND.) The young woman's comment made my day, and it is likely one of the nicest things anyone has ever said to me.

Marcel LaPerriere

I hate ALS more with each passing day and know things could be much worse. My life is full of too many blessings to count. ALS sucks, but life is good. No, life is great!

Familial ALS

17 July 2018

My sister-in-law, Carol, sent me a text in early May telling me that my brother Jay, ten years my senior, might have ALS. That sparked many questions and emotions. Like me, my brother is confined to a wheelchair. Jay has been suffering from COPD for the last four years, and about two years ago he started having problems walking. About a year ago he could no longer walk at all. At first his doctors thought his loss of walking might be due to Parkinson's disease, but in May, they told him it was not Parkinson's and it was likely MS or ALS.

Jay is now in the "wait and see what happens" mode. More tests are planned, but the tests take time to schedule, perform and return results. Jay and Carol are now waiting to see what happens with more tests and more doctors' visits. And, I, of course, wait too.

Ever since I heard that Jay might have ALS, I've wondered if we both have familial ALS, or if we both have sporadic ALS? What is the chance that two siblings would have sporadic ALS, since ALS is so rare? Then again, familial ALS is even rarer, with only about 5 to 10% of the 5600 people diagnosed with ALS in the USA annually having the inherited version of the debilitating disease.

The big question: was there any ALS in our family's past? Carol, Jay and I all agreed that there didn't seem to be any on our father's side of the family. But, what about our mother's side? That is where the trail would lead. Or so we think. We don't know much about our mother's father. That grandfather was our grandmother's second husband, and our mother was born well after our grandmother already had and raised children. By the time our mother was born, her siblings were all in their teens and twenties. None of our mother's three step-sisters developed ALS, and two of the three sisters lived well into their 80's. Our grandfather was in his late 50's when our mother was born, so we know nothing about his siblings or any of his ancestors. Could any of them have had ALS? If they did, that would have been in the 1800's, so no one knows? Since our mother died young, we must wonder if she died before she had a chance to develop ALS. Again, we just don't know.

The haunting question since Carol sent that text is, if it is familial ALS, did I pass on the ALS causing genes to my son and he to his sons? And did my siblings pass on the genes to their kids and their grandkids? Connie and I asked my neurologist if I should be tested to see if I carry the gene, or genes. She said, "Wait and see what the outcome of your brother's tests are." She went on, "You already know you have ALS, so the more important question is, does your son or his children have the gene, or genes. Please, keep in mind that just because they might have the gene or genes, doesn't mean they will develop ALS. It only means they are more likely to." She continued, "When you know about your brother, if he does have ALS, then you need to tell your son. It would then be his decision to be tested or not. Until you know, there is no need to worry your son." I haven't said anything to my son, and that is bugging me. Should I tell him about Jay and the possible ALS? Ugh. I don't want to worry him or his wife, but it's tearing me up not sharing this information with him. I wish my brother's medical diagnosis wasn't taking so long.

Now we wait, and as we wait, I worry. I can't do anything about what genes I have passed on, but if I have passed on the ALS gene or genes, I will be fraught with guilt. How could I not be, knowing what a terrible disease ALS is? I have read where other people feel guilt for passing on troubling genes to their kids. But is this justified guilt? There could never be an easy answer to that question. It is very sad to me to think I might have passed something bad on to the very people I love.

Marcel LaPerriere

Too Late

21 July 2018

Recently I have been looking though boxes and albums of old photos. After I had looked at hundreds of photos, my cousin Michelle, whom I hadn't seen in fifty years, came to visit us here in Alaska. Because she is such a nice person and because we have a shared lack of information about our families, she wanted to see some photos that I had recently been going though. She got to know a little bit about Connie and me when I shared

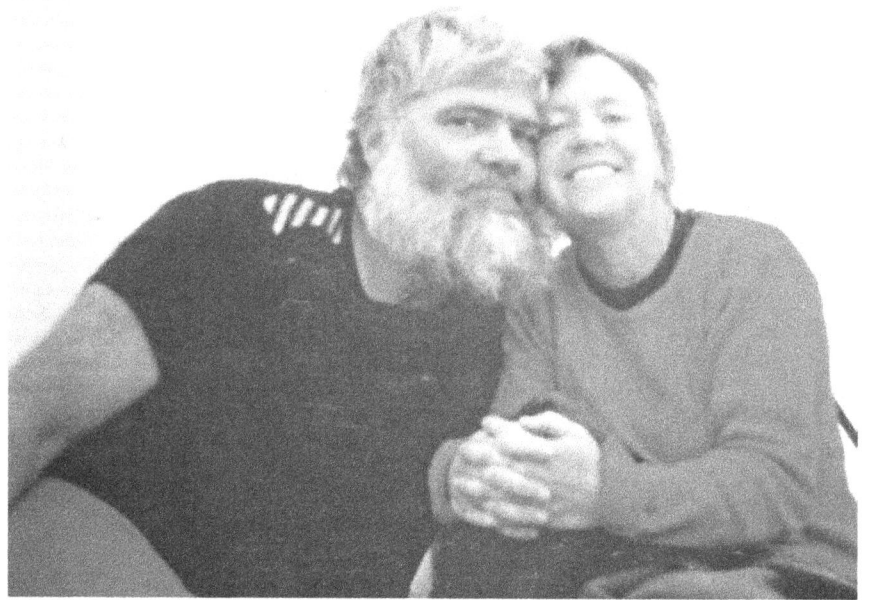

2000. After a week of hiking and no showers, Connie and I wait in our tent at Grace Lake for the boat that will transport us back home.

the photos with her. Plus, we both learned more about our fathers and their families. Our fathers were brothers, and even though they were somewhat close, Michelle and I knew little about each other or other mutual relatives.

Not only did we gain knowledge of each other, but I got to relive many adventures Connie and I shared in the 46 years we have been together.

One thing that struck and even surprised me was how many fun adventures that we have shared. Of our photos of family, sailing, canoeing, caving, climbing, backpacking and travel, without exception, the photos of Connie and me together brought back many fond memories.

Before Michelle arrived, when looking at some poor-quality prints of one of our backpacking trips, I remembered what a fun time we had. Even though the photos were poor quality, that was one of our best adventures. I typed into my phone for Connie to read, "I sure wish we had done more of these trips." She made some comment about how it was too late now, and I nodded, "Yes." Then I typed, "In our next life, we will know to make more time for fun and adventures." Were it only that simple to live another life to correct our mistakes.

The mistake most of us make is thinking there will always be time later to do the things we want to do. Then we get busy with jobs, raising a family and the other distractions of life. We quickly justify not taking the time or spending the money for those things by saying, "Later." Though we had many fun adventures, we still found way too many excuses to put off what we really wanted to do. Work, a new truck, house payments, or some other excuse often stopped us from another adventure. Those things seemed more important, and I'm not saying they weren't. But, in retrospect, all those excuses didn't build the memories that I now cherish.

I had no control over when ALS would hit and then rob me of abilities to do the things I so loved doing. What I did often control was how we prioritized what we did and when we did it. Both Connie and I way too often said, "We will do that someday later."

The main reason I'm writing about regrets of not doing more fun or meaningful things is that I hope others can learn from my mistakes. If you are saying things like, "next year, sometime in the future, after we retire," or a whole host of other excuses, please keep in mind that "later" might not come. Connie and I often talked about all the things we would do when we retired. Little did we know that just when we reached the cusp of our retirements, that whammy of ALS would hit me. With 20/20 hindsight, it could have been any health issue that got in the way. I thought bad things happen to other people, not me. I was in good shape for my age. At 60 I was still out-hiking people half my age. I had never smoked, almost never drank alcohol, ate healthy organic foods, got plenty of exercise and got plenty of sleep. Yet a health issue stopped me from doing what I wanted to do.

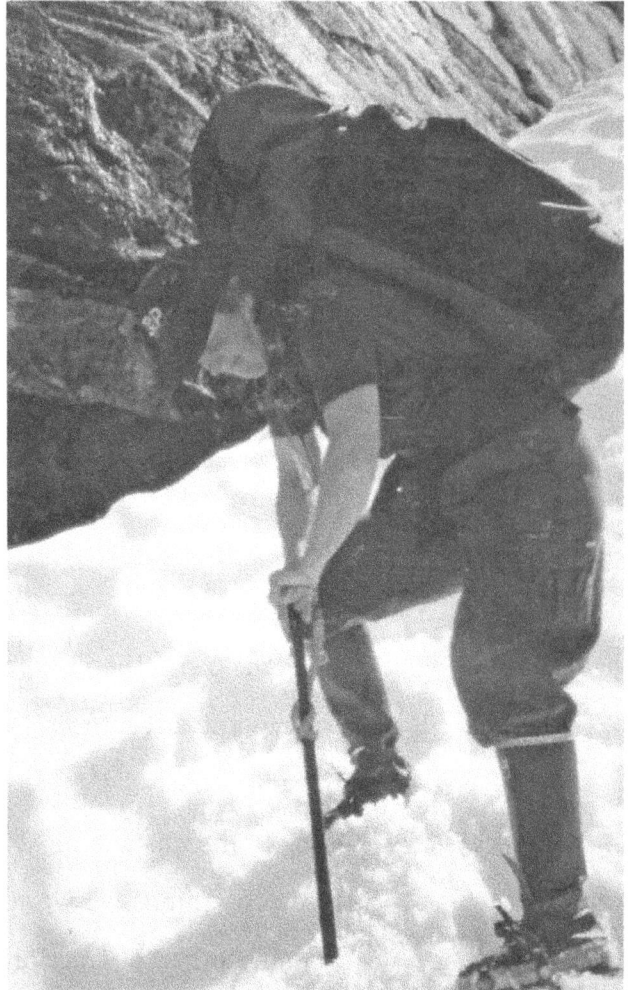

2000. Connie —— off-trail hiking in Misty Fjords National Monument.

Although we didn't do a fraction of the things I had hoped to do in the Adventure Department, we still did more than most Americans. As I sit in my wheelchair writing this, I can look back on many fond memories that help me ward off the blues. Take the backpacking that I mentioned. On that trip we flew by float plane into a remote Alaska lake, then hiked for a week in country that has seen few, if any, human feet. The second day, as we walked along an alpine ridge, we ran into a large herd of mountain goats —— of the forty-some goats that we saw, none had ever seen humans before. The fourth day, as we hiked in heavy fog along a knife edge ridge near the summit of very remote peak, Connie exclaimed in a surprised voice, "Look —— a dog. What the heck is a dog doing up here?" Looking over her shoulder at the animal a few feet in front of her, I said, "That's not a dog, it's a bear." Yes, a small black bear –– small enough that I wondered where its mother was. Because of the heavy fog, we back tracked and let the bear pass. On the second-to-last day of the trip on an old abandoned logging road, walking towards our rendezvous with a boat that would take us the thirty-eight miles back into Ketchikan, we once again ran into a bear. This time it was a very mature and very large black bear that didn't want to yield to us. Our only weapons were ice axes in our packs, so, we followed what all the books say to do: we raised our arms in the air, we made lots of noise and we stood our ground. When the magnificent bruin walked off the road into heavy brush and let us pass, we watched him with a little trepidation –– he was also watching us. After we had passed him, he walked back onto the road and continued his journey.

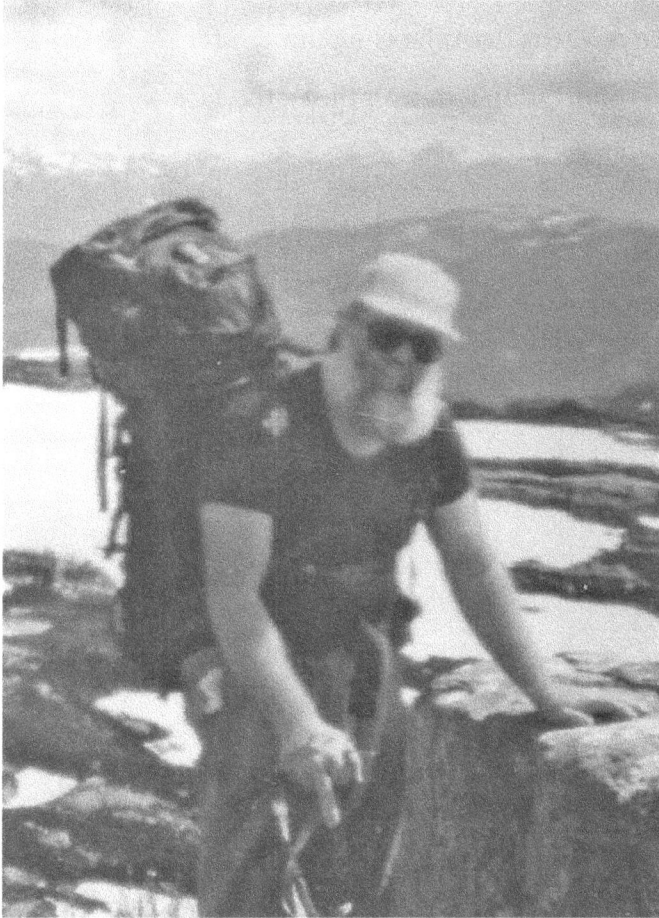

2000. Marcel with an 80-pound backpack.

I'm lucky to have many adventures to look back on as well as memories that revolve around family, which is a good reminder of the importance only family bonds can bring. As long as I live, I'll try to add more good memories to the memory bank. A big thank you goes to Michelle and her daughter for traveling from the east coast of America to Alaska. Their trip will add assets to my memory bank, assets more valuable than the money that I have in the bank. Sometimes it takes an illness to learn that memories from life experiences are what makes life worth living. An old friend often said to me, "Money –– it's only paper." How right he was. Paper doesn't last, but memories do.

Before it is too late, make some memories to add to your own memory bank. Unlike withdrawing money from a bank, when you withdraw memories, they go right back in and pay much bigger rewards than the compound interest on your money investments. Life is too short; don't wait until it's too late for you, too.

Emotions

31 July 2018

The other day my sister-in-law, Carol, and I were exchanging a few text messages, and the emotion of hope came up. I texted her that there is no cure for ALS -- so any hope that I might have is false hope. But I also said, "Just because I don't have hope doesn't mean I'm not happy and enjoying life." Later, I wondered if I sounded too flippant, and I hoped not. That also started me thinking about a whole host of descriptive words, including the word, "hope."

Just because I don't have hope that I'll get better doesn't mean that I'm not hoping for a cure for ALS. However, I'm also realistic enough to know that any cure for ALS will come too late for me. That doesn't mean that I'm not hopeful that a cure will be found. Neurological diseases like ALS are extremely complicated, which means any cure is likely many years, if not decades, away. That doesn't mean I'm not hopeful for better therapies to help people live longer and improved lives. There are several drugs that show very promising results, and that gives me hope. And there are many more promising drugs just on the horizon. Therefore, I'm also very hopeful that those drugs will become available soon.

Marcel LaPerriere

More about descriptive and clarifying words. Some of the negative words that popped into my head were bitterness, depression, pity, frustration and animosity. I've seen how bitterness in a person living with a progressive disease can lead to depression and self-pity. I've then seen how frustrating it can be for those who live with the sick person, and I've seen how that can build animosity. So, I'm grateful that, other than frustration, I have mostly warded off the other negative emotions. And, I hope that bitterness, depression and self-pity never creep into my disposition. Keeping negativity at bay is not always easy, and I hope to keep enjoying life, even as my ALS progresses.

Some of the positive descriptive words that came to mind: happiness, family, love and laughter. I'm extra lucky to have a family that I love, and I'm even happier that we often laugh together at silly things. All my grandsons have a good sense of humor, and they make me laugh with their wit and silliness. Also, our little dog not only makes me laugh every day but brings us such joy.

I may not have hope that I will ever get better. But I'm happy and in love with the same gal I've loved for over 46 years. Therefore, life is good. Life might not always seem fair, but even with ALS I'm living a better life than many other people around the world. So, why would I be bitter about not having hope? ALS is just another journey that I may not have chosen, but one I can live with. Despite ALS, I can live life with happiness and joy. The decision of how I choose to live life is mine, and I'll do what I can to keep the negativity away and to choose positive emotions over negative emotions.

Obstacles

2 August 2018

The old saying, "You need to walk a mile in the other person's shoes before you can understand," could be changed to, "You need to spend a day in a wheelchair before you can understand." I had little understanding of all the obstacles that a handicapped person faces before I ended up in a wheelchair. The last six months have been a real eye-opener for me.

I'll start with public restrooms. Have you ever noticed that in many restrooms the handicapped stall is all the way at the far end of the restroom? In one of the Seattle airport restrooms, it's almost as if someone said, "Oh, we almost forgot. We need to add an American with Disabilities Act (ADA) stall." So, at the end of ten or twelve toilets, they throw in the ADA stall. At the time I needed that stall I was still using a walker. Since I can't talk, imagine what it was like for me to nudge my way through the extra full and busy restroom. Now, imagine what it must be like for a person in a manual wheelchair. To me it's appalling. Shouldn't the handicapped stall be the first toilet you come to as you enter the restroom? And, please save the handicapped stall for people who need them. All too often, I've seen perfectly healthy people come out of the handicapped stall when there are other stalls available.

Marcel LaPerriere

Even in our small town, I've had some less than desirable public restroom experiences. In our community center, the new restroom has a button to open the door. Recently when I went to use that facility it was closed for cleaning, so I wheeled down to the older restroom. That restroom has no button to open the door. Have you ever tried to open a heavy metal door while sitting in a wheelchair? If you have, you know it's not easy. I thought that door was challenging until I tried to open the door to the men's public restroom along the Seawalk. Not only is there no button on that door, but due to some maintenance that was done last winter, the sidewalk was dug up and not replaced. As I tried to roll over the rough gravel, I had to open the door and then try to hold it open while wheeling myself over a three-inch lip to enter. By the time I did get into the restroom I had over-exerted myself to the point that I was nearly puking. Then, even though there is clearly a handicapped sticker on the sign for the restroom, my chair did not fit into the stall. That posed a problem that I'll skip telling you about. By time I did get to the toilet, I'd nearly peed my pants.

Now that I have a power wheelchair I'm finding a whole new set of obstacles, like no curb cuts, overgrown brush crowding sidewalks too narrow for my chair, cars parking on the sidewalk, cars blocking the curb cut, power poles placed in the middle of the sidewalk and more garbage cans than I can count. Then there was a guy walking his dog who refused to step off the sidewalk. And a guy riding his bike at breakneck speed down the sidewalk. Just a few feet before he would have run into me, he jumped his bike off the curb and onto the road where he should have been in the first place. Or curb cuts so steep that I drag the foot pegs and, as I go off the curb, the rear wheels of the chair lift off the ground for a second or two.

A most annoying obstacle is someone standing in the middle of the sidewalk, talking or texting on his phone, totally oblivious to his surroundings. This happened to me twice yesterday. Since I can't talk, and my power-chair is so quiet, getting his/her attention is the problem. The horn on my chair is quiet and not very effective. Since my chair and I together weigh 610 pounds, I don't want to go off the sidewalk and onto the wet grass, for fear of getting stuck or worse. I sat there for about a minute just a few inches from the person, until at long last he saw me and moved. He didn't apologize or make any acknowledgment that I was even there; too, wrapped up in the phone conversation to notice or care.

More annoying than the cellphone zombie was a very large pile of fresh dog poop right in the middle of the sidewalk. As I carefully avoided getting dog poop all over my chair's wheels, I wondered how people can ignore the fact that their dog has pooped all over the sidewalk and then not clean it up? Maybe it was the guy who I saw just a few minutes before that didn't want to step off the sidewalk with his dog?

I'm learning many things I never thought I'd have to learn. But I'm grateful that my eyes have been opened to what life is like for a handicapped person. I'm also grateful for the people who stood up for handicapped rights and forced the US Congress to enact laws like the ADA. Without these activists in the 70's and 80's, venturing out in public would be much harder, if not impossible. I applaud those civil rights pioneers and thank them for helping make life a little easier for those of us who are handicapped.

Marcel LaPerriere

Baching it

5 August 2018

While Connie is in Seattle for surgery to fix a bunion on her left foot, Bella and I have been baching it this past week. We're not much good at it, so are anxiously waiting for Connie to return home. Bella has been suffering full-blown separation anxiety. If ever there was a dog that shows full-on depression, it's Bella, and she has been mighty sad wanting her momma. The first two nights that Connie was gone, Bella lay under my nightstand and cried herself to sleep. Unlike Bella, I'm happy Connie has gone south to have the surgery that will keep her doing what she loves to do –– hiking. After Connie's foot is better, Bella will be happy too –– she just doesn't know it. Bella is Connie's inextricable hiking partner. The two of them have almost become conjoined hiking buddies. Connie's foot pain was getting to the point that the pain was so acute, it was taking away the fun. It was time to have surgery, and Bella will be happy that Connie had it fixed. Meanwhile, we both are missing her greatly.

Late last February, when we were in Seattle for some of my medical appointments, we visited Dr. Heit, a podiatrist at Virginia Mason Hospital, about Connie's bunion. Her bunion stuck out like a sore thumb, or in this case a sore toe. The X-ray that Dr. Heit ordered brought home how bad it was, and

44

it was soon clear to both of us surgery was the best option. Dr. Heit didn't push surgery but pushed for less invasive measures. He told us that many people live for years with bunions, something we knew because Connie had already been doing that. He told us some serious runners will go years with bunions and that they either use orthopedic inserts or cut a hole in their shoes to make room for the bone deformity. With the preferred hiking footwear for our wet climate being Xtratuf rubber boots, cutting a hole was not a viable option. And Connie had already been using custom-made inserts in her shoes and boots for several years. It was time for surgery.

Besides not wanting to ruin her summer hiking, Connie also was concerned about taking time away from her other duties to have the surgery. The two duties she worried the most about were not being around to walk Bella and being my primary caregiver. To me, that's one of the under-appreciated things about a caregiver; it's hard for them to take time off for their own medical needs. On the other hand, I knew that Connie's daily walks and her longer hikes are the ways she unwinds. Therefore, I did all I could to encourage her to get her foot fixed. We both knew that with ALS, the responsibilities of the caregiver increase as the disease progresses. We decided that early August was the best time for her to have the procedure done. That way she'd still get in most of the summer hiking, and the timing should be good for asking others to walk Bella. Not to mention, if my ALS gets worse, which it almost for certain will, then being gone at a later date wasn't going to get any better.

It's not been easy not having Connie here to help me with all the things I depend on her for, but I'm managing. It helps that Connie pre-made me several dinners and froze them, so all I need to do is throw them in the microwave. I'm lucky that most everything I need I can reach while sitting in my wheelchair. With my son, Zach, or my grandson Blake stopping in to walk Bella, I have someone I can ask to do other things that I can't do.

Marcel LaPerriere

Other than missing Connie, some of the simplest things have been a little challenging, like unloading the dishwasher or the clothes dryer. I can reach both while sitting in my wheelchair, but a task like putting dishes away that used to take me under five minutes is now problematic. When sitting in a wheelchair, that task is now taking around twenty minutes. No big deal, I just put on a podcast, put a clean dishtowel on my lap, stack a few dishes at a time on my lap and then wheel myself to where they need to go. It's slow, but it works. Perhaps the hardest task is giving myself liquid though my PEG feeding tube. That task requires three hands and sadly I don't have an extra appendage. Reaching things is also challenging without help. For instance, there was a box of dog treats that I needed to get that were under the clothes-folding table in the utility room. As hard as I tried I just couldn't reach them from my chair. Dare I get down on my knees, and if I did, could I get back up? I wasn't sure that I could. A couple of months prior, while putting on some pants, I had forgotten to lock my wheelchair wheels, which caused to me fall onto the floor, and I had gotten back up that time. But could I do it again? Since I had my cell phone in my pocket, I figured if I couldn't, I'd call Zach. When he saw it was my number on his caller ID, I figured he'd come check on me. Or I could text one of the neighbors. Worst case, I'd text Connie and ask her to call the Sitka Fire Department to help lift me back into my chair. Though it was a little scary, I lowered myself to the floor, grabbed the box, and with a little bit of difficulty was able to get back into the chair. Mission accomplished, and with the box of treats in hand, there was a happy little dog to reward my efforts.

I now have even more appreciation for people who face being handicapped on their own. I couldn't help recalling a video I saw a few months ago of a woman with ALS who lives on her own. She not only PEG-feeds herself all her meals but was still taking public transportation to her full-time job. The video didn't say what she did for work, but she sure has my respect.

Being alone this last week has reminded me how lucky I am to have Connie as my wife. And, even though Bella can be a real pain in the rear when she gets me up three or four times during the night to go outside, I appreciate that cute little dog to keep me company. I also appreciate the help from my family and neighbors. I owe a big thanks to my neighbor Christine for walking Bella today.

Time to go do the juggling act of PEG feeding myself. I just hope I don't spill prune juice all over myself. I hate being sticky, and prune juice is just that.

Gimp

12 August 2018

When you look up "gimp" in a dictionary you will get several meanings, including a flat trimming of silk, wool, or other cord, sometimes stiffened with wire, for garments, curtains, etc. "Gimp" is a derogatory word to describe a handicapped person or a person with a limp. The word "gimp" is only derogatory if used with malice –– I often call myself a gimp. And, with Connie temporarily wearing an air foot-splint and an exoskeleton leg brace after her foot surgery, in my loving eyes, she too is a gimp. If "gimp" is used in a hateful way, it's wrong. But it's okay if used to lighten the mood when talking about a person like me.

Yesterday we were trying to come up with a name for our new handicapped accessible van. "Gimp Mobile" didn't seem all that

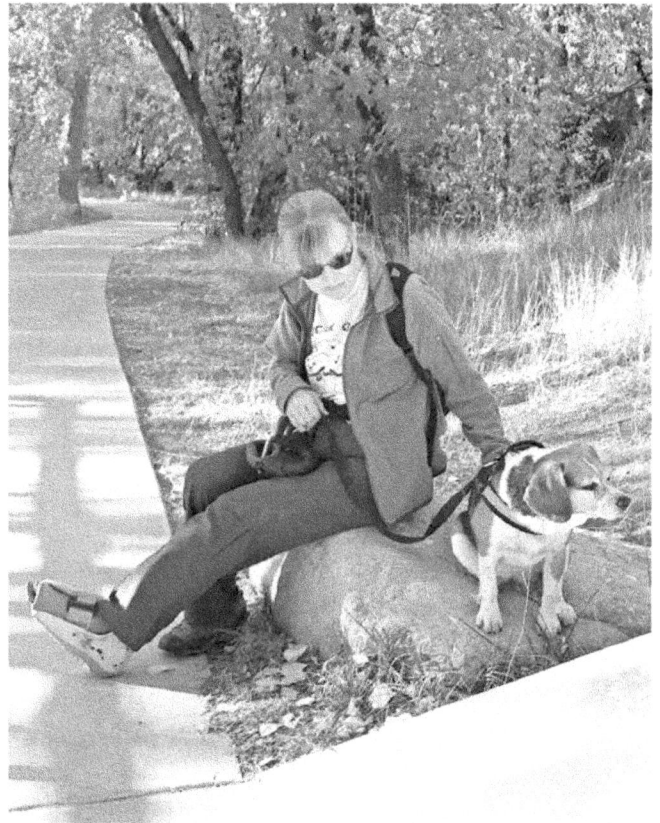

September 2018. Connie and Bella on a walking path along East Plumb Creek, Castle Rock, Colorado.

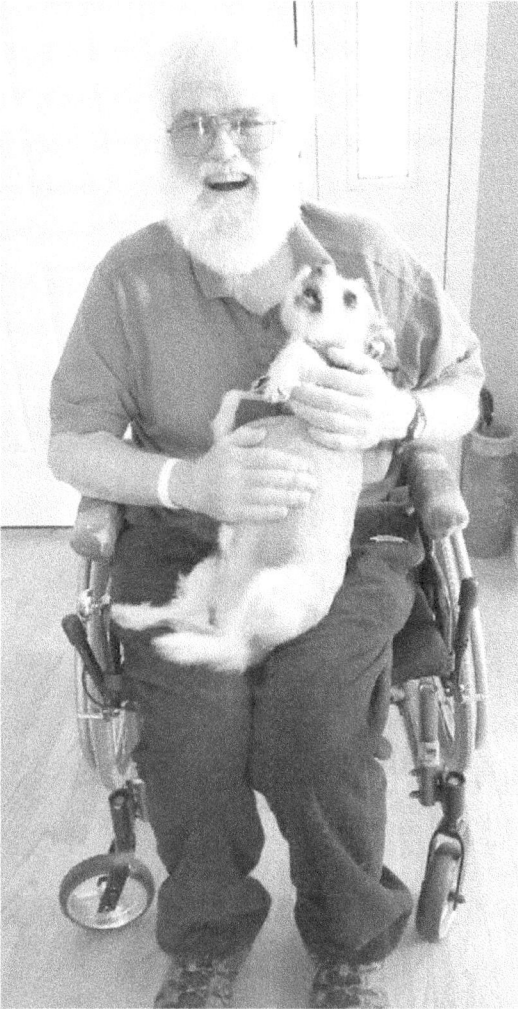

September 2018, Castle Rock, Colorado. As I rolled into my sister, Andree's house, her little dog, Wile. E., greeted me by jumping into my lap.

original or creative. Since we both like puns, we considered "Van Haulen," a play on Van Halen. When you listen to their song "Jump," with its catchy tune, then "Van Haulen" seemed like an okay name. It was nixed because Connie thought the song "Jump" might be too catchy, and we would constantly be humming it every time we got into the van.

I then though of another pun, "Gimp-en Van Go." But, the van is a whole unit, and so far, not missing an ear or any other parts. So, maybe that name isn't right either? Or is it?

At this point we will just have to see what sticks. We really don't need a name for the van, but, now that I'm dependent on not only the van but a power wheelchair, I'd like to add some levity to the situation. Humor has helped me deal with what is otherwise depressing, so, for now the van is "Gimp-en Van Go." That's until something else hits our fancy and helps us laugh at the fact the we are both "gimps." I'm glad Connie is just a temporary "gimp," but, since I'll always stay a "gimp," I want to keep some laugher and humor in my life, as I face living with ALS.

Marcel LaPerriere

The ALS Association

18 August 2018

The ALS Association in recent days has been taking some flak from some of my fellow sufferers of ALS because, according to their 2017 IRS form 990, they are sitting on 96.4 million dollars. Looking at one year's 990 is like a doctor basing a decision on your health just by looking at your body temperature. Just like I want a doctor to look at all aspects of my health, you need to look at the complete picture of the ALS Association.

Let's look at the 990's going back to 2008 and see the financial trends.

Cash on hand:

2008	7.9 million
2009	9.5 million
2010	13.8 million
2011	17.5 million
2012	17.5 million
2013	17.5 million
2014	20.7 million
2015	119.7 million
2016	104.4 million
2017	96.4 million

50

The trend shows slow and healthy growth from 2008 to 2014. Then, because of the great success from the Ice Bucket Challenge, the cash at the end of the fiscal year 2015 jumped by 99 million dollars. Since the big jump in 2015, the cash is slowly going down. Their financial picture over a ten-year span shows good management. Also, it is highly unlikely that the ALS Association will experience the kind of growth they did in 2015, which also shows good financial planning.

A more important number is the ratio between administration and program granting. They grant out 81% of the money they take in. Compare that to any other nonprofit and you will see why Charity Navigator gives them a score of 96.48 out of 100.

We all want a quick cure for ALS, and we'd all like to see more money spent on research. I just don't want to see one of the primary worldwide fundraisers for ALS research throwing money out the window. As a person who has given and will continue give money to the ALS Association, I'm glad the information that I can garner looking at their 990's and from their non-profit ratings show they are doing a darn good job.

It's easy to be a Monday morning quarterback sitting in the wings wanting a quick cure for a disease that we know will kill us. Having sat on many nonprofit boards, I know from firsthand experience that the hardest mission of any nonprofit is figuring out the budget and how to most effectively spend money. I also know what it's like to be saddled with not enough money to do the things that the nonprofit was set up to do. Or the headaches that can be passed on to future boards when previous boards make bad decisions. The ALS Association should be given a big hand of applause for their obvious good job of raising funds, building a lasting nonprofit organization, and for the vital funding that they have supplied. Their ten years of data shows that they are in it for the long haul. That is what will be needed if there is ever to be a cure for probably the most complex of all the neurological diseases.

Marcel LaPerriere

No one will gain if they spend their fund foolishly. Thank you, ALS Association, for the fine and important job that you are doing.

Maladie de Charcot

22 August 2018

"What's ALS?" is a question that I wasn't overly surprised to hear from a delivery truck driver. But when I hear it from a person who works in the medical field, I'm always a bit surprised. Just last Monday when we went to see my primary care doctor, a new nurse in his office had a mighty confused look on her face when Connie said, "Marcel can't talk because of ALS." As the nurse started taking my vitals, she asked Connie, "So what's the underlying problem?" Connie again said, "ALS." The nurse then asked in a confused voice, "What's that?"

I haven't kept track, but in the last two years, between phlebotomists, radiology technicians and nurses, we have been asked, "What's ALS?" close to a dozen times. Even a doctor who was doing rounds in a hospital asked, "Isn't that Lou Gehrig Disease?"

I'm not sure when I first heard of ALS, but in the early 60's, as a grade school kid, I had some understanding of what Lou Gehrig disease was. Lou Gehrig was long gone by the time I was a kid messing around on the baseball field, but we boys who loved baseball revered him as a hero, just like we revered Babe Ruth or Ty Cobb. Even though we had no idea what a neurological disease was, we held Lou Gehrig in higher esteem than other baseball stars because we knew he had bravely faced his own death from a disease that was so rare it was named after him.

In the early 90's I read Stephen Hawking's book "A Brief History of Time" and thought about the terrible disease he was living with. I admired his work and his brilliance –– being able to do complicated math just in his head. I also admired his bravery, living with such a devastating disease. If even a non-medically educated person like me knew about ALS, how can a person who works in medicine not know about it? Or give Connie a look as if she was talking to them in some alien language? To be only a little silly, when Connie said, "ALS," the nurse looked at her as if she had said, "grumfenug trabotten barfragell."

Given all the media coverage of the Ice Bucket Challenge, how can anyone still ask, "What's ALS?" If I could talk, I might jokingly ask, "Have you been living under a rock these last few years?" ALS is a relatively rare disease, but shouldn't you know what ALS is? If you work in the medical field, you should not have to ask, "What's that?" There is still a lot more work to be done on the ALS awareness front.

So, What IS ALS?

26 August 2018

A few people have asked me to explain what ALS is, so, here goes. ALS is different for every person who has the misfortune to experience it. Also, I'm not a medical expert. Everything I write is either something a doctor has told me, something I've read, or something from personal experience.

ALS stands for amyotrophic lateral sclerosis. In the United States ALS is also often called Lou Gehrig Disease, because the baseball player from the 1920's and 30's who contracted the disease in 1939 was famous, and the disease was so rare. Lou Gehrig appears to be the first celebrity to suffer the malady, so his name just stuck to the disease. In the rest of the English-speaking world, ALS is called motor neuron disease (MND). That name describes exactly what ALS is –– a disease of the motor neurons.

ALS was first identified in 1869 by a French neurologist named Jean-Martin Charcot. Charcot, the Father of Neurology, was also the first doctor to identify multiple sclerosis. Even more interesting, he studied with Sigmund Freud and others who laid the foundation for modern psychology. The French name for ALS is, not surprisingly, Maladie de Charcot. When we traveled to France in 2016, I put that name on the medical alert bracelet I always wear.

First, nearly everyone asks if there is a cure for ALS. The answer is no. Next, they ask, "How long will a person live with ALS?" Though hard to answer, worldwide statics say from two to five years. That said, Stephen Hawking lived with the disease for over 50 years, and I have heard of one person who succumbed in five months. I have no idea if there were other underlying health problems with that person.

ALS doesn't discriminate between races or gender, but it is slightly more prevalent in men. The average age when it strikes is 60, but there are rare cases when it has been diagnosed in teens as young as 15 and in the elderly over 80. ALS also tends to be slightly more prevalent in people of European descent. Also, for some unknown reason, if you are a military veteran, you are twice as likely to develop it compared to the civilian population. In the US, there are approximately 30,000 people living with ALS, and there are around 5,600 new cases per year. The least common type, about 5 to 10% of the total cases, is called familial ALS, which means it is inherited from either the mother or father's side of the family. All other ALS cases are known as sporadic ALS, which means that there is no known reason that the person has developed it.

Preliminary data shows that NFL players are also much more likely to develop ALS, with an estimated 42 cases within retired players over the last few decades. It's assumed that NFL players are more likely to develop ALS because of head trauma, but that is speculation. There also seems to be a higher number of ALS cases in professional soccer players –– again, possibly because of head trauma.

Back to motor neurons. Basically, motor neurons are the communication wires that lead from the brain to the muscles to tell them what to do. There are two types of motor neurons: the upper motor neurons, which are in the brain, transmit to the lower motor neurons in the spine. All forms of ALS are the breakdown of the motor neurons. Though way above my knowledge level, I'll make a stab at what researchers think might be the cause of this breakdown.

Other than familial ALS, which researchers know is caused by the genes one inherits, it's thought there might be a gene mutation that causes the motor neurons to not function properly. This could also be caused by a chemical imbalance, the body's gradual accumulation of abnormal proteins, or possibly the body's own immune system attacking healthy nerve cells. Or it could be a combination of the above, or something else.

No two cases of ALS are alike, yet there are obviously similarities. In most people, ALS starts with muscle fasciculation, which is just a fancy way of saying a twitch, followed by ever-increasing muscle weakness, until the muscle no longer functions. For some people these symptoms start in a finger. For some, a leg, or arm, or in my case my tongue, and throat muscles. Death is most often caused by the diaphragm muscle no longer being strong enough to support breathing.

I fall into the approximate 25% category of what's called bulbar onset ALS. Bulbar onset strikes the brainstem's corticobulbar area, where the motor neurons are that control the tongue, neck, head, and facial muscles. That is why bulbar onset ALS affects the voice and swallowing. Since those motor neurons control facial muscles, that's why I can no longer talk or pucker up to kiss my wife. Something as simple as blowing on hot food is impossible. Plus, my facial muscles under my beard have sagged, could you see them. Smiling is impossible. When I open my mouth as wide as possible, there will be a hint of a smile.

Another frequent question is, "Does it hurt?" Again, not an easy question to answer. Not being able to talk physically isn't painful, but, since we humans are social animals, yes, there is an emotional pain associated with not being able to talk.

Marcel LaPerriere

The literature on ALS says there isn't much pain associated with ALS. I'll call BS on that. Almost everyone who has ALS will experience severe muscle cramps and charley horses that often hit while sleeping. I had bad cramping in my leg muscles, sometimes hitting both legs simultaneously, and sometimes cramps would also hit my arms. No matter where they hit, they hurt like hell. Since I've had ALS, I also have a lot of joint pain. How would a person not have joint pain if the muscles that hold the joints together stop working? I've also experienced muscle strains and back strains from something as simple as rolling in bed. And the inside of my mouth usually looks like raw hamburger because my facial muscles don't work, which causes my checks and lips to sag inwards. That means I'm going to bite them. I find this to be especially a problem at night when I have my bilevel positive airway pressure (BIPAP) ventilator mask on. The mask pushes my lower lip up to my teeth, and if I bite down, I take a chunk out of my lip. There is physical pain associated with ALS.

Since the most complex organ in the animal kingdom is the human brain, it stands to reason that a neurological disorder like ALS is also going to be very complex. When you couple in two relatively new medical studies, the study of the human microbiome and how it effects the human body, and the study of human facia tissue, the equation gets even more complex. Does the facia tissue that runs the full length of the spine play a role in ALS?

Science now knows there are over 10 trillion bacteria cells living in our bodies, which means bacteria out number our own cells by a factor of 10. Do those cells contribute to ALS? When I consider the complexity of the disease, I see why one of the first neurologists I saw, a woman doctor from an Eastern Bloc country where they are used to adversity, told me she thinks a cure for ALS is still 200 years away. I hope she is wrong, but she obviously has a more realistic view of how complex the disease is than I do.

Maybe this analogy will help us better understand diseases like ALS. Since humans first looked up into the sky and saw birds flying, they wanted to also fly. Now, consider a modern airplane and all the systems that are required to make it fly. Dozens of systems requiring tens of thousands of parts all need to work together to get the plane off the ground. No one human can understand every part and system that makes the plane fly. Yet, somehow it does. It does because of teamwork between many different specialties all coming together with the common goal of doing something that on the surface looks impossible. I think the cure for ALS will be much the same in reverse. No one person will ever truly understand how the brain works, and how it integrates into the whole body and all our complex systems. It will take many teams from many different disciplines to come up with a cure for ALS. That's why I'm happy that hundreds of labs and medical professionals from around the world are working on this very complex puzzle. A worldwide database that is now possible because of the World Wide Web might be the ticket to a cure.

Jerky Convulsive Movements

27 August 2018

Lately I've been having a lot of jerky convulsive movements in my legs. It's hard to describe, but here goes.

Without warning, my leg will do a sudden jerk followed by very rapid convulsions. This usually happens when I'm asleep, or just falling asleep. Also, just as the process starts, it often feels like my leg has been electrically shocked –– there is a feeling of a shock, followed by a large jerk and then the convulsion of my leg or ankle that lasts just a few seconds.

Last night these jerky convulsions were happening every five to ten minutes. I'd just fall back asleep and they'd happen again and again. Also strange is that the involuntary movement range and speed is greater than my voluntary abilities.

Postscript: I posted the above on the British Facebook site, "MND Warriors." Within minutes, many other people said they too suffered from this same thing. The advice was to take magnesium, and I've started doing that. It seems to help, and the convulsions have been much less frequent.

How Much Longer?

2 September 2018

Yesterday, while I was cruising down the Seawalk in my motorized wheelchair, I ran into an old acquaintance. As he approached, he greeted me with, "Hello," followed by, "How are you doing?" Since I long ago lost my ability to talk, I waved and gave him a "thumbs up. As he came alongside my chair that I had stopped, he asked, "Is this your new normal?" I nodded, "Yes," to which he asked, "So, how long will you need to use a wheelchair?" This caught me off guard, because I know he knows I have ALS. Since I couldn't verbally answer, I typed into my phone, "Forever." That was quicker and easier than what first came to my mind. I had wanted to type, "Until I die, which I hope is a long way off." As he walked away, he said, "That's too bad, but at least you're getting out for a walk." And how right he was with that parting comment.

      I'm still often amazed at how little people know about MND/ALS. My friend recognized the importance of getting out of the house. It helps me feel more normal. Besides, I do love getting out and about town.

Medical Vacation

3 September 2018

Tomorrow we leave on a two-month road trip vacation. I'm looking forward to the trip with excitement and trepidation. Excitement, because a road trip though the Western United States is always fun, and we will see lots of family and old friends. Trepidation, because we book-end both ends of the trip with medical stuff in Seattle. A week from today, Connie will have her post foot surgery follow-up and will be instructed how to transition to walking using that foot. We expect everything to go well. The anxiety comes over my doctor's visits and what that means, not only for our road trip, but our future.

Just because a person has a rare disease like ALS doesn't mean that other health issues are put on hold. Blood work shows several of my hormones and my prostate PSA levels to be out of whack. My primary care physician, Dr. Hunter, wants me to see a urologist and an endocrinologist at the Virginia Mason Hospital. Since my ALS journey started with a diagnosis of acromegaly and the removal of a benign tumor on my pituitary gland, that might or might not explain why so many of my hormones are out of balance. Often with acromegaly, even when the tumor has been removed, the patient still experiences hormone imbalance problems. And, like many men my age, prostate problems are to be expected.

Experience tells me that one visit with a specialist always results in more tests being ordered, then more tests and more visits with the specialist. Thus, it is nearly impossible to stack appointments close together. So, while we are waiting between tests and doctors' visits we will road trip. The uncertainty of test results and follow up appointments makes it darn hard to plan where we will be going and when we will get there. A major goal is to get to Colorado to meet one of Connie's cousins and her husband from Florida who will be in Colorado mid-September.

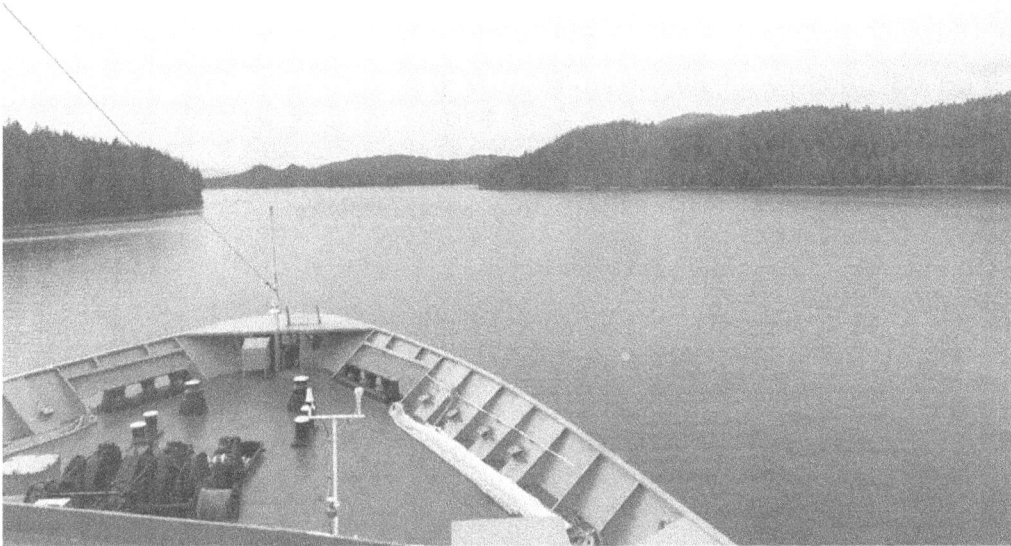

The other yin and yang is the start of our trip with a 57-hour, 800-mile trip on the Alaska State Ferry. We love that trip through some of the most beautiful inland waterway passages in the world, but we know it's hard on our little dog Bella. Dogs, un-

September 2018. The view from the observation deck on the Columbia ferry, cruising through the Inside Passage in British Columbia, Canada.

less they are service dogs, must stay in the vehicle with limited ability to get out and walk. We will stop in three other ports during the first 24 hours of the trip, so Bella will get to walk and do her business on land. It's the other 33 hours through British Columbia when Bella will get very limited walks on the car deck. She will not do her business on the car deck. We have tried every trick in the book to get her to, but she refuses. So, she does it in the car. Even though she makes a mess that we must clean up, it's okay with us, because we feel so bad for her. Leaving her home is not an option either. She loves road trips and she loves being with us. Connie and I have debated whether the ferry trip is harder on Bella or us, because we feel so bad for our little dog. In the past I have literally cried when we had to lock her in the vehicle for another leg of the trip.

During this trip we face a couple of new challenges. This will be the first long trip that we have done when I'm confined to a wheelchair. That means that Connie will be doing all the driving. And, unlike me, she doesn't like to drive for endless hours. Also, we will need to find hotels that will take dogs and have handicap accessible rooms. Fortunately, more and more hotels will take dogs, and unless we get way off the beaten path, we should be able to find hotels that can accommodate me and my wheelchair.

Knowing that ALS is relentless and will continue to progress, this is likely our last vacation and road trip. This could also very well be the last time I see some of my family and friends, my birth state of Colorado and so many other places that Connie and I have grown fond of. Even with those sobering thoughts and the unpleasantness of medical visits, we will endeavor to have the best time we can and enjoy life to the fullest.

The Ferry Columbia

5 September 2018

Yesterday, as we boarded the Alaska state ferry Columbia, I was transported back in time to 1973. Connie and I arrived by Greyhound bus in Seattle during the waning hours of 1972, just in time to welcome in the New Year with less than $40.00 in our pockets and nothing in the bank. We were flat broke. We needed jobs, and the quicker the better.

New Year's Day 1973 fell on a Monday, so Tuesday the 2nd saw us both out looking for jobs. We had already scrounged the two Seattle daily newspapers off the waiting room seats in the bus station, and one of the ads was for a welder working at the Lockheed ship yard, located on Harbor Island just south of the main Seattle port. Lockheed was building the Alaska state ferry Columbia. I had a little welding experience and three years of high school metals shop, so I applied for the welding job. During this time unemployment in Seattle was off the scale because Boeing Aircraft Company had lost some big government contacts. There were billboards on the outskirts of Seattle that read, "Will the last one out of Seattle please turn off the lights." It was not a good time to be looking for a job in the Northwest.

Marcel LaPerriere

Even with the odds stacked against me, Tuesday morning found me knocking at the front gate of Lockheed, filling out an application and taking a welding test. I failed it miserably, and I'm extra glad I did.

At that time in my life, the biggest boat I had ever been in was a pedal boat for rent on the City Park Lake in Denver. So it was exciting for a 19-year kid recently out of high school to be walking through a big shipyard. I can still see the molten metal from a cutting torch and the sparks from an arc welder cascading off the hull of what would become the Columbia, giant cranes swinging large sheets of steel right over my head, and forklift trucks carrying loads while they did what looked like a choreographed dance, weaving in and out of buildings. I was totally entranced with all the goings on when I saw the building that I was to take the welding test in.

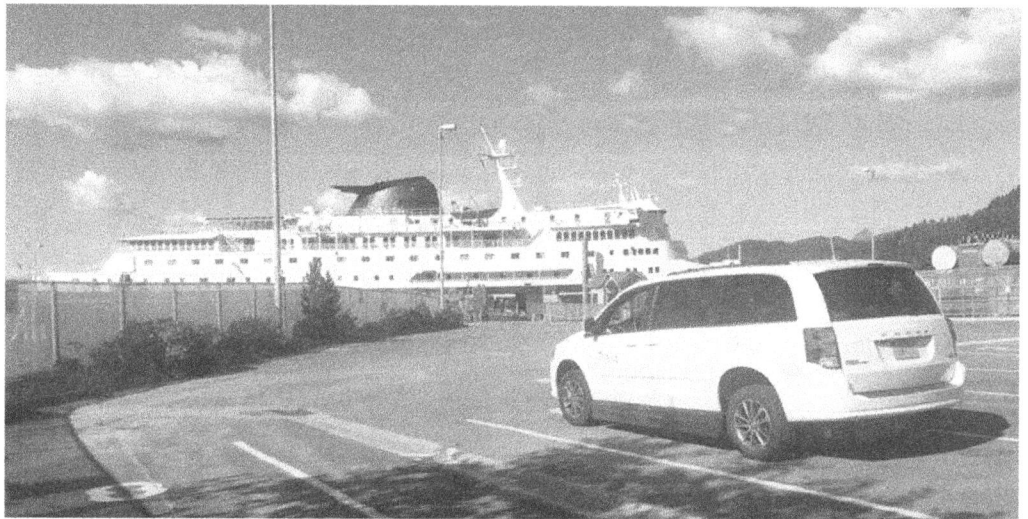

September 2018. Ready to board the Alaska State Ferry, Columbia, in Sitka, Alaska.

It was a very typical and dirty welding shop with all the assorted stuff you'd expect to see. When I told a very friendly middle-aged man I was there to take a welding test he directed me to a welding booth and handed me two chunks of steel I was to weld together. The two chunks of steel were about half an inch thick, by three inches wide, by six inches long. On the width, a 45-degree bevel had already been cut, and that is what I was to fill with weld until the two parts became one. The nice man said, "You'll find an assortment of welding rod over there, and there is everything else you will need in the booth." It surprised me when he then said, "To set your amperage, you will find the controls on the welder that sits on the roof. Take the outside stairs up and find the welder that is numbered the same as the booth you will be using." Who had ever heard of a welder sitting on the roof of a welding shop? I sure hadn't.

I picked welding booth 4, grabbed some 6011 and 7018 welding rods, set them on the bench and then headed for the roof where I saw the oldest, largest and the most worn out welders I'd ever seen. There were six welders about 2 1/2 feet in diameter and about 6 feet long. Each welder was lying length-wise on a heavy-duty steel pipe stand, and sitting on top of the cylinder was a large box about two feet square by a foot deep. On the front of the box were two large rheostats for adjusting the amperage. One was a course adjustment, and one was for fine tuning. Both took what we called "Armstrong tuning," to turn the knobs. You had to be darn strong to turn them.

It took a couple of trips up and down the stairs to get the amperage where I wanted it. But even with that delay I had the two pieces of steel married together in just a few minutes. When I took my sample weld to the inspector, he took one look and said, "Nice looking weld, but I can see it's not very strong. Let's test it and see if I'm right." With that, he put the test piece in a machine that would stretch the weld until it broke. After putting both ends of the steel in some jaws that gripped it, he closed a heavy metal screen door and then turned the machine on. I watched the gauge slowly and steadily climb, when suddenly, "BAM," it broke. Unclamping the two chunks the inspector said, "Just as I suspected. It broke at about half of what it should have. The mistake you made was trying to weld it with too few passes. See how it broke on the weld? If you had done it right with six to eight beads, grinding each weld, then, instead of it breaking on the weld, it should have broken on the edge of the weld, taking some of the virgin metal with it." After chatting a bit more about what I had done wrong he said, "I'll tell you what. If you want to take the test again, come back in a week and we can try it again." I said I hoped to have a job by then, and he again offered me the same opportunity if I wasn't lucky securing a job.

By the time a week had rolled around, I was working a dream-come-true job as an apprentice machinist for the Hallidie Machinery company. That apprenticeship laid the foundation for every job I worked thereafter.

But I wasn't done with the Columbia. Before the Columbia had even hit the water just a few months into my new job, Hallidie got the job of repairing the brand new babbitt bearings that the Lockheed workers screwed up when sandblasting sand in got in the propeller shaft bearings. Dirt and sand don't mix with that super soft metal used in babbitt bearings. Hallidie's employee, Bob Hale, was an expert on repairing large babbitt bearings, and he needed some special tools to execute the repairs. I'm the guy who made those tools, which are probably still in some Alaska state repair facility, because they were unique to repairing the Columbia propeller shaft carrier bearings.

Bob not only had an expertise that few people have, but he was a heck of a nice guy. A gentle giant of a man, he stood 6 foot 4 inches, wore size 15 shoes, and was built like a linebacker. During my apprenticeship, he taught me a little of what he knew, always showing compassion and treating me like one of his own sons who by chance were my age. By coincidence, when we moved to Ketchikan, it was Bob Hale Jr. who gave me my driver's license test. And Connie worked with Bob Jr.'s wife for several years.

A couple of other times at Hallidie, we did small jobs for the Alaska Marine Highway system. At least one other time I made a part for the Columbia, so she brings back a few nostalgic memories.

Though I didn't get the welding job, I did more than my fair share of welding over the years. Maybe my ALS was caused by all the welding fumes I breathed in? I was much too cavalier when it came to working around toxic welding fumes. So, now that my grandson Blake has taken up metal working and welding with a passion, I harp on him every time I get a chance. I don't want him to make the same mistakes I did. And I sure as hell don't want him to ever have ALS or any other disease that can be prevented by protecting his lungs. So, Blake, when you read this, please take my advice and every other safety warning I've given you.

Ferry Day One

5 September 2018

Really, night one.

The ferry Columbia gets a failing mark for handicapped accessibility. I don't mind the small elevator, but on every deck, one needs to go up a ramp to access the lift. The car deck is the worst. I could never have made it up that ramp in my wheelchair without the help of a very friendly Alaska Marine Lines employee. The other decks also have ramps, but I can get up them okay.

The supposed ADA (Americans with Disabilities Act) room accommodates my manual wheelchair only if I take off its foot rests, and it is nearly impossible to get it past the head [toilet], which has a large bump for a threshold. It's very tight, and the bump obstacle is encountered while trying to make a 90-degree turn. Once in, the grab bars are so low as to be almost unusable.

The camber on the deck makes it hard in a manual chair. From port to starboard, first one must climb up the radius, and then once amidships, it's a wild ride down the other side of the camber. When going the length of the ship, the camber pulls the wheelchair towards the outside of the ship. I can live with the camber; it just makes it more of a challenge. It's the thresholds that are monster obstacles to get over.

The Adventure Continues

The Columbia is one of two Alaska state ferries that have real dining halls and not just a cafeteria. I'm delighted to give them high marks for good food and service.

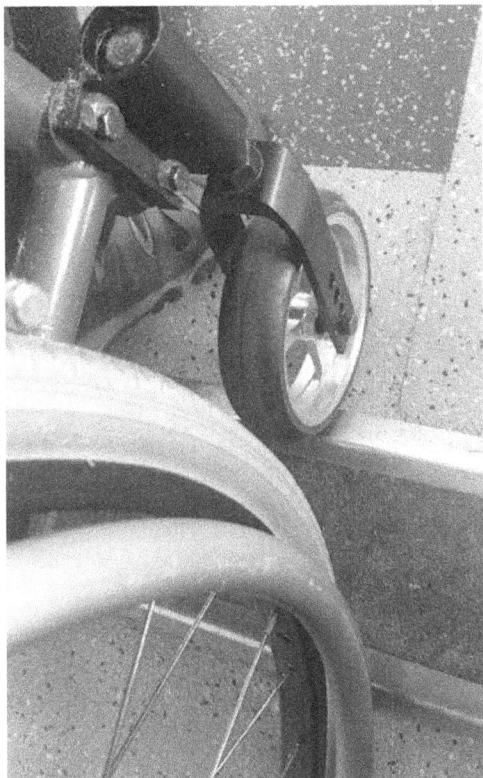

September 2018. The threshold wheelchair traps that are ever-present on the Columbia.

We could not get the key to open our stateroom 207, so Connie got the Purser, who also failed, but moved us to 209. Since 209 had the head all torn apart, we were back to 207. Even new keys wouldn't work for 207. The solution: don't lock the door.

The beds on the Columbia are bunk beds. No joke. Connie, with her healing foot, had to climb a ladder to the upper bunk, knee, foot, knee, knee, foot. And me getting into the lower bunk was a task pushing my limits. There is nothing to grab onto, the overhead bunk gets in the way, and the angles of approach are all wrong. On boats, a bunk or bed is often called a rack. In our supposed ADA stateroom, the name rack fits. I wondered if it had been designed by the Spanish Inquisition, it was that uncomfortable. I'm sitting in my wheelchair at 4:00 am because I couldn't take it any longer. I was starting to hurt on top of the sore spots that were on top of the hurting areas. The ferry system should market these rooms to sadists. Who knows -- that might be a viable market?

The Columbia was built 15 years prior to Congress enacting the ADA and has undergone several major renovations since 1990. They totally have failed meeting the intent of the law as far as staterooms. When we return home in a couple of months, we hope to be on one of the other ferries, one that hasn't failed as badly as the Columbia has.

Even with the obstacles of traveling on the ferry, we are still having fun. Now, back to the rack for a couple of hours of torture.

Marcel LaPerriere

Booking a Handicapped-Equipped Room

8 September 2018

Our education continues. This will also sound a little like an endorsement of the LaQuinta hotel chain.

One of my main reasons for posting what it's like to travel when you're confined to a wheelchair is so others can learn from our mistakes.

This will be our fourth long road trip in the last four years. Of the dozens of hotels we have stayed in over a combined six months and close to 40,000 miles of driving, we have found the best, most consistent dog friendly hotel chain to be LaQuinta. We feel we always get the best value from LaQuinta —– the rooms are always clean, and the service always comes with a smile.

This time we sort of got let down by LaQuinta. We booked an ADA room online, and when we showed up for two nights in the Bellingham LaQuinta, we did get a "sort of" ADA room. When we arrived, we were told that LaQuinta policy requires a phone call to get a full ADA room. So instead of a roll-in shower we got a tub. Because they have excellent grab rails, and I can use one arm to lift my legs while the other hand holds onto the grab bar, I'm going to take advantage of a tub and take a bath. I haven't had a sit-down bath since we moved to the 1st floor in our house several months ago, so I'll enjoy it. We now know that online booking for a handicap room doesn't cut it.

Live and learn. Plus, I say go with the flow. When a mistake is made, make the best of it.

Post Bath:

Did you ever look forward to a nice dinner out with your sweetheart, only to go to the overpriced restaurant and find the food only mediocre? Or spend all day looking forward to finishing that nice chocolate cake you baked a few days ago, only to find that in the cake was now dried out and stale? My long-awaited sit-down bath was much the same.

I made it into the tub without too much difficulty. Washed my hair while standing, and then figured I'd have a nice long soak. Getting down in the tub proved harder than I thought, and when I sat down it hurt like crazy. I no longer have any padding, so it was the metal bath tub against my bones. To make matters worse, my breathing has become so compromised that the warm moist air was hard for me to breathe. I was beginning to think Connie would have to call the rescue squad to lift me back up. After several minutes of struggling, I managed to roll onto my knees and pulled myself up enough to sit on the rim of the tub. A couple of minutes and a lot more butt pain later, I managed to get back on my feet. Lesson learned –– I won't do that again.

Beds

13 September 2018

One of the biggest challenges one faces when traveling as a handicapped person is the various beds. There is often not enough room to get a wheelchair properly placed to make the transfer from chair to bed and back. But the biggest challenge for me is that the head of the bed isn't elevated. At home I use a hospital type bed, and elevating the head of the bed makes it easier to breathe. In fact, without my BIPAP ventilator I'd be in big trouble. As ALS progresses and the diaphragm becomes weaker, it helps to sleep with the head slightly elevated. Also, with no elevated head, there is nothing to grab onto to aid when getting in and out of bed or even rolling on my side. I'm near my limit when I roll onto my side.

Speaking of sleeping on one's side, I learned something the other day that has been helpful. In my daily news feed there is often a health suggestion. Often it's of little use to me –– for instance, I have no use for suggestions on how to safely remove mascara. But the suggestion the other day was to sleep with a thin pillow between your knees when sleeping on your side. The article said it helps align the spine to reduce back pain. It sure has worked for me.

The one thing I'm enjoying about hotel beds is that I'm in the same bed as my wife and our little dog, Bella. When we got Bella in April 2014, Connie said, "There is no way a dog is sleeping in our bed. Period." That lasted about two weeks, when a very cute little puppy put her front paws up on the bed, looked at us, and in the most pathetic little cry let us know she wanted to be in bed with us. Even though it often means a paw in the face or a dog snoring in our ears, we love a snuggling little dog in our bed. With my hospital type bed at home, Bella never makes the step from Connie's bed to mine. So, it's been special when a little puppy comes over and snuggles up next to me. In spite of me tossing and turning the other night, Bella kept snuggling closer and closer.

There have been some challenges, but also some benefits sleeping in a different hotel bed each night. The experience of traveling is worth the effort.

Marcel LaPerriere

Super 8 Hotels

28 September 2018

So far on our road trip across the western United States, the most user-friendly handicapped rooms have been in Super 8 Hotels. They're basically cookie cutter designed, with few modifications hotel to hotel. Also, I have met one of the men who started the Super 8 chain. Since his roots came from small town Middle America, where he was much more likely to rub elbows with farmers and ranchers than three-piece suit business men from Wall Street, practicality is not a surprise.

Below is an excerpt from a very long short story I wrote about a Chevy Blazer my brother, Fred, owned for many years and then gave to me.

> It must have been 1998 when we decided to leave the Blazer in Whale Pass on Prince of Wales Island, Alaska, and use it as an island car. One day, out of the blue I received a call from a filming crew that said they had permission and the proper permits to do some filming in the caves on Prince of Wales. They asked if I could take them around and show them caves that they could access from the road. Mostly they were interested in filming a cave dive or two. When I said I would take them around, they told me the owner of the filming company would be in town in a few days along with the cave diving stars of the documentary they planned on filming. They said the owner would be flying his

helicopter and it was arranged that he'd fly us over to the island and then I'd drive them around in the Blazer, which was parked at the public dock in Whale Pass.

The owner of the company was a self-made man who had made his money starting one of the largest hotel chains in the US. After he sold off most of his hotels, he went into a sort of semiretirement and started a company that did documentary films around the world. He'd travel to the filming locations in his fancy extra-large power yacht, fly his private jet, or in the case of the Prince of Wales Island caving documentary, he came to Alaska in his private Bell Jet Ranger helicopter. Bright and early on Saturday morning, which was one of those glorious sunny days with no wind that can bless Southeast Alaska on rare occasions, we took off from the Ketchikan Airport. Since the weather was so beautiful, I was in for a flying treat unlike none I'd ever experienced, though by this time I'd flown in a helicopter hundreds of times for work. After taking off and flying to the north end of Gravina Island, he then decided to fly over Clarence Straits about five to ten feet off the water at a cruising speed over 130 mph. At one point, he buzzed a small boat with two guys that were out fishing, flying just feet above their heads. I could easily see that his flying antics had scared the living you know what out of the fishermen, but it sure made the maniac pilot smile. When we arrived at the island, he flew on to Whale Pass at an elevation that was just a few feet above the tree tops, all the while flying over 100 miles per hour. Landing in Whale Pass was also a bit of an adventure because there wasn't a whole lot of room at the dock, but he managed to find a place to set down and we then transferred from the flying racing machine to the good old Blazer.

The night before this mini-adventure, the owner of the filming company had taken Connie and me out to one of the nicest and most expensive restaurants in Ketchikan. As we ate dinner, we made plans and talked about the caves we would visit. As part of the planning, the owner said that he'd swing by the store in the morning and grab us all lunches. Now, keep in mind this man is a multi-millionaire, or possibly a billionaire. After all, he not only owned the helicopter that would take us to Prince of Wales, but he also owned another helicopter, a half dozen planes and at least one business jet. And, that doesn't count his large yacht that had a crew of around 15 people. So, when he said he'd pick up lunch and that it would be his favorite food for lunch, I was of course, expecting something extra fancy. Well, imagine my surprise as we put the tailgate down on the Blazer, and started to make lunch. My jaw dropped all the way to the ground as he started by pulling out a loaf of Wonder Bread®, then a box of Kraft American Cheese®, French's Mustard®, a large bag of potato chips and cans of warm Pepsi®. All food that I'd never eat. I did eat it, and even though it wasn't the caviar that I had expected, I was hungry enough that it tasted good.

(The documentary was titled, "White Rock, Blue Ice." Unfortunately, it was not all that good.)

Party Line

29 September 2018

In my youth, "party line" had a completely different meaning than it does today. When I was a kid, a party line was referring to the type of phone service we had. This is going to age me, but for those of you who don't know what a party line was, please let me tell you.

Back in the day of rural telephone service, before technology made it possible to carry more than one conversion on a phone line, you'd often have to share your phone line with several families in the same neighborhood. In our case we had an eight-party line. There were the Kobes, the Parrishs, the Harrisons, the Walters and four other families all sharing the same phone line. Each family had a unique ring, so when the phone rang, you'd listen to hear if it was your ring, and if it was, you'd answer the phone. If you were making a call out, first you'd pick up the phone and listen to be sure that no one else was on the phone. If the line was clear, you'd dial the number you wanted to call or call the operator. If you wanted to call someone that was on the same party line, you'd dial the number, hang up, wait for the phone to ring, and once you heard it stop ringing, you'd then pick your phone and say, "Hello." This system worked well as long as you didn't have a phone hog on your party line. The other fallback was people on the same phone line could "listen in" on your conversation. And, if truth be known, from time to time almost everyone listened in. This was before cable TV, and even FM radio was rare, so "listening in" became a pastime for some, entertainment for some, and a full-on obsession for a select few.

Mrs. Walters was on our party line. Not only did she listen in on conversations endlessly, she also wrote the gossip column in the local weekly paper. In fact, my siblings and I were often featured in such important news as, "Marcel got a new pair of shoes for school and Andree a nice new dress." Or, "Fred has been breaking his horse, Ziegler, and is making good progress. His goal is to have the horse ready to help Joe Kobe with the fall roundup."

I'm writing about party lines because now that I have ALS and can no longer talk, I often feel as if I'm just listening in on others' conversations. Just the other night at dinner, Connie, my sister and brother and their siblings started talking about the old party line and how our mother got to hate Mrs. Walters for invading our privacy. As I enjoyed listening to the conversation, it dawned on me, that's what I was doing: just listening in. And, instead of a gossip column, I now have access to social media where I can post to a worldwide audience.

As my ALS continues to progress, and I lose more and more dexterity in my fingers, listening will become an even bigger part of my life. Some months ago, a woman who I think uses eye gaze technology to communicate, posted that to her, ALS was one of the loneliest diseases she could imagine. She said before ALS, she loved having long conversations with friends, and now, because it's so hard for her to communicate, she basically only communicates essentials. I'm not at that point yet, and I hope I never am.

As I lose the ability to move my hands and fingers, communicating will become a bigger challenge. It's already tough enough, so I'm not looking forward to that. However, I'm going to continue enjoying just listening into my fellow humans as they carry on their conversations. I don't know if I'll ever use eye gaze technology to talk, but it's nice knowing that it's out there if I do need it.

Not being able to talk is both frustrating and a bit lonely. But I'm lucky to still be alive and still enjoying life. As we road trip across the western United States, I appreciate having a wife I love and such a great extended family. As much as I hate ALS, I still love life each and every day.

Technology

2 October 2018

I have a love-hate relationship with technology. On one hand, I depend on my iPhone for several things, including talking. On the other hand, the frustration with devices that don't work right can be maddening.

Take the Garmin GPS in our van. Why does it always direct us to a freeway when it's often quicker and less maddening to take an off-freeway route? Or today when we entered Winnemucca, Nevada, I searched for nearby restaurants, and it gave me a Dairy Queen a few hundred miles away in California. Then, when it did give a local restaurant, all it showed was a Jack in the Box and not the half dozen other fast food or other restaurants. And when I punched in nearby parks, it gave me a park in Oregon.

I find the GPS in my phone that uses Google Maps much more reliable. But my carrier, AT&T, doesn't work in Winnemucca. That's funny, because I had good cell service when we were in the middle of nowhere –– but when we got to the first decent sized town after five hours of driving, no cell service.

Speaking of phones, just before we started this road trip, my speaking app would from time to time stop working. Not wanting to buy a new phone, I decided to see if I could live with it or fix it. It soon became obvious that I needed the talking function so that I could communicate with Connie. One Apple store, two AT&T stores, and about five hours of frustration for Connie later, I got a new phone. But within a few hours, the speaking app was not working again. Ugh. Seven hundred-fifty dollars and several hours of transferring everything to a new phone sent me back to Google to search for a fix. After reading several articles and watching a couple of videos, I stumbled into an obscure hint that it might be caused by the Bluetooth option. Eureka! With the Bluetooth off, the app no longer crashed. I never would have guessed that, because I've used the Bluetooth option for a few years in our Toyota truck and our Bose Sound System. So it's something with the Bluetooth connection in our new Dodge van. Who would guess that an automobile would cause a phone app to crash? I sure wouldn't have.

One piece of technology that I've been very happy with is my new power wheelchair. So far it has performed flawlessly. And, the battery life is much better than expected.

My love-hate relationship with technology will continue. And, I'll keep scratching my head each time the GPS sends us to a restaurant two states away.

Marcel LaPerriere

Trophy Wife

6 October 2018

As I lay awake, trying to sleep on one of the most uncomfortable hotel mattresses ever, my mind drifted back almost thirty years. On our sailing schooner Terra Nova, we had already lived aboard the semi-finished 45' on-deck steel hull, bouncing from temporary stall to temporary stall within the Ketchikan, Alaska, Bar Harbor Marina for over three years. At long last we got a permanent stall. That stall was on Dock 8, and we were mostly surrounded by commercial fishing boats. On our side of the dock were the larger seine boats, and on the other side of Dock 8 were gillnet fishing boats and trollers. One well maintained troller named Lady May, was owned by an elderly couple that fished more from long-standing habit than from necessity. We didn't personally know the owners of the Lady May but they were always friendly, and I could tell they were dedicated to each other and their fishing boat.

Shortly after we moved to Dock 8, our son, Zach, who was a senior in high school, was selected as an exchange student, and he left for New Zealand for a year. Connie and I knew that with Zach gone, we would have a perfect opportunity to focus on finishing the interior of Terra Nova. So, if we were not at work, we were slaving away on the boat interior with no time to socialize with our new neighbors. That changed when a very good shipwright named John from New Zealand, who was circumnavigating the Pacific with his wife, Jean, in their boat, Sinu-K-Tam, tied up their boat for the winter, right across from our slip, on Dock 8.

I couldn't believe our good fortune in having a fully qualified and very talented shipwright literally docked just across from Terra Nova. I can now admit we paid John cash under the table to help us work on the boat. He was glad to have an infusion of money for their cruising, and we were glad to have a skilled craftsman to help us with our massive job.

Not only did John help, but we soon became good friends with both him and his wife, and we often ate dinner together. At one of those dinners, they told us that they had met Bob and Kitty, the owners of the Lady May, and had been invited to dinner at their house. Right after that dinner we were told that Bob thought I was a "dirty old man married to a trophy wife." Both Connie and I found that funny. In defense of Bob, Connie had always looked much younger than she truly was. Yes, I'm older than Connie, but she is far from being a trophy wife, unless a year and a half younger qualifies her for that title. In further defense of Bob, more than once people thought Connie was Zach's sister and not his mother. And, even crazier, I was once accused of being Connie's father. So Bob can be excused for thinking I had a trophy wife.

Though wrong about Connie's trophy wife status, if he were still alive today, I'm sure he'd agree that Connie deserves a trophy for her dedication to being my caregiver. This was especially true as we traveled our way across several western states. Not only did Connie have to do all the driving, but pretty much everything else as well.

My day normally starts at 5:30 or 6:00 am. I'm still able to roll myself into the shower, and I normally do that while Connie catches a few more zzz's. Once out of the shower, I don the clothes Connie has laid out for me, and she gets up and gets us breakfast. After we eat, Connie makes three trips to pack the van for the day. Then it's time to walk Bella before we hit the road. Throughout the day Connie will walk Bella a few more times, get us lunch, check us into a hotel for the night, and then make a trip to a store or restaurant for our dinner. I haven't mentioned that each time I get in or out of the van there are four tie-downs for my wheelchair that need attending to. I can't even help when she stops to get fuel. So, while I basically do nothing more than take up space, Connie does all the work. I feel safe in saying when Connie said, "I do," after the part about "for better or worse," she had no idea what she was signing up for. There is never a bitter word from her, and she just marches on. Yes, she deserves a trophy, if for nothing else, making this a fun vacation.

I'll back up now and tell you that we became good friends with Bob and Kitty. There were many things we liked about them, but two things about Bob stick in my mind. For one, he was brutally honest. When we'd go over to their house for dinner, Bob would often say, "Well it's time for you to go and for me to go to bed." This was usually about two minutes after the last bite of food. The other thing we always enjoyed was Bob's word of the day. Each day he'd randomly pick a new word out of the dictionary and then use it throughout the day. Sometimes he'd have to be very creative. For example, "The king salmon seem to be experiencing a diaspora. We sure aren't catching any, so they must have been displaced from their home spawning area." We also loved hearing about the bar in Ketchikan they owned and many fishing stories.

Bob passed away like all of us want to –– after mowing their small lawn, he came inside for a nap in his lounge chair and just never woke up. Kitty was, of course, devastated, as we all would be upon losing a spouse after fifty-some years of marriage. She surprised us all when she moved to Port Angles, Washington, to live with their daughter. Even more surprising, she met up with and married her old high school boyfriend. Both were in their 80's at the time, and both had lost their first spouses. We got an occasional letter from her for five years or more until one day we heard that dementia had gotten the best of her.

John and Jean finished their circumnavigation of the Pacific and made it home to New Zealand. They continued to cruise the waters of the South Pacific for many more years until age and failing health forced them to sell their beloved boat and take up land cruising in an RV. While John kept busy in his woodworking shop, Jean wrote a book about their sailing years, called *The Tiller Years*, by Jean Porter.

Life is full of twists and turns that none of us can ever predict. I might not have been lucky falling victim to ALS, but I was sure lucky to have Connie as my wife. And, I feel blessed to have experienced many things that give me such good memories. As age or health issues stop us from doing the things we used to do, all the good memories help ward off the blues. My advice for the young generation is be sure you are building good memories. Live life as if there is no tomorrow, and do everything you can to foster happiness.

You Look Good

12 October 2018

"You look good," is a phrase I hear often from both friends and family. They are right –– I do look good and healthy. Aside from having ALS, I'm in fairly good health. But, I'm far from good. No one with advancing ALS can be considered to be in good health.

One given with ALS is there will always be more and more declines. What's not given is the timing of that decline. There could even be small improvements. At least in my case, the improvements never seem to last much more than a couple of weeks. ALS is different for everyone. There are no two cases exactly alike.

As we approach the six-week mark of our road trip vacation, I've noticed that despite the fact we are having fun, my decline is marching on. I'm having a harder time standing, transferring from my power chair to my manual wheelchair, getting in and out of bed, and even getting off and on the toilet. I also continue to lose dexterity in my fingers. Simple little things like grabbing a single napkin out of a stack is now a real challenge. And tying my shoes is also a challenge –– I must lift my legs up onto a stand with my arms to reach my shoes.

The saying goes, "Getting old is not for wimps." That applies double for ALS. Another saying goes, "It beats the alternative." That is true for both getting old and ALS.

I hate the continued decline caused by a neurological disease that I have no control over. But I do control my attitude dealing with facing a disease that will continue to steal abilities from me. As the ALS Monster continues to take, I will not let it give me bitterness, depression, anger or any other negative emotions. It scares the daylights out of me, but I'll live life as fully as I can each and every day. I'll take, "You look good," as a compliment. Then, do my best to look good inside.

Mileage

21 October 2018

When I was a kid, a story about someone who owned a car that got unbelievable gas mileage went something like this. "I know a guy who knows a guy whose uncle owns a Ford Galaxy that gets over 50 miles a gallon. Ford made a dozen cars that got mileage like that and then destroyed them because the oil companies paid them off. One car somehow got missed and ended up being sold. It's my friend's friend's uncle who owns that car." Of the several versions of the story –– sometimes it was a Chevy or a Chrysler –– they all told of the unbelievable gas mileage.

I own the power wheelchair that has unbelievable battery life. When I was being fitted for the chair, the salesman said, "The factory says the battery life is good for 12 miles." At the time, I thought, "Yea right." He then clarified it by saying, "That's on flat ground with no load." So I was expecting maybe six or seven miles before I needed to charge the battery. The other day I went 17.7 miles and still showed 40% battery left. And the next day I went 8.5 miles and only used 35% of the battery. Yesterday I put 6.7 miles on and used 25%. Even better, today when I turned on the wheelchair power, it showed I still have 90% of the battery left.

The Adventure Continues

I'm the lucky guy who got the prototype, Permobil f3 Corpus that has unbelievable battery life. So if you hear about some guy who knows some guy who owns a wheelchair that has a battery that lasts and lasts, I'm that guy.

Eyes

23 October 2018

I ignore the progression of ALS until it slaps me in the face and I am forced to acknowledge yet another decline. This time the ALS Monster is making it hard for me to see. ALS doesn't cause a person to go blind, but the muscles that move my eyelids are weakening. That means I can't open my eyes as wide as I used to be able to, and when I blink, it is what I'd call a lazy blink. The blink is slower than normal, and my eyes don't totally close when I blink.

It's now time to hit the Internet and see what I can find out about this malady. I've only heard of this eye problem in one other ALS patient, and that man had to tape his eyes shut to sleep. It's worse in my left eye, and I always have a big bag under that eye.

As scary as it was to lose my ability to talk or walk, losing my ability to see is even scarier. I won't be happy if I can't see. But I'm not going to get depressed over it either. I'll continue to fight off negative emotions as the ALS Monster continues to make me face things I'd just as soon not be facing.

Last Vacation

1 November 2018

Connie says I shouldn't say it, but I'm 99% sure we have just returned from our last vacation. Two months on a road trip has taught me that traveling is not easy when you have a progressive neurological disorder. I hope I'm wrong, but I need to be realistic, while still being positive.

In spite of the many obstacles to traveling as a handicapped person, we had fun. It was likely more fun for me than Connie because she had to do all the driving, most of the associated work, care for Bella, our beloved little beagle, and me.

The other day a friend asked us what the highlight of the trip was –– I said seeing friends and family. We also lucked out experiencing a two-month-long display of fall colors. As much as we love living in Southeast Alaska's abundant rain and fall wind storms, fall colors usually don't last very long. So being immersed for two full months in the brilliant, yellows, oranges and red colors was truly a gift.

I'm extra glad we made the trip. Though we spent a large portion of our son Zach's inheritance on it, I wanted to make a few more memories with the gal I've loved for over four and a half decades.

Marcel LaPerriere

If I have any advice for both the healthy and those like me that are living with a fatal disease, it's to make the most of each day. Spend as much time with friends and family as you can. Experience the giving and taking of love. And, most important, live life as fully as you can. Do all you can to make as many good memories as possible. Do that each day and you will have few regrets in your waning years.

Progress and Progression

5 November 2018

It's interesting to me that the word "Progress" is most often used to connote something positive –– whereas, the word "Progression" is often used to describe something that is not positive. I can't consider progression of my ALS a good thing. If I add two little letters to the word "Progress" to make the word "Progresses," which suggests forward or onward movement, when describing my ALS, it's not a positive thing.

The one given with ALS' progression is that it will always bring new losses and challenges. As I type this, I'm challenged by that progression on three fronts: my eyesight, my finger dexterity and my ability to breathe.

Because I'm now having a hard time opening my eyes all the way, I'm now looking though my eyelashes. That makes it hard to position my eyes in the right position to properly use my bifocals. This decline has taken me by surprise, as the eyesight decline is not generally considered a symptom of ALS.

The lack of dexterity in my fingers is much like when one's hands are cold –– they seem stiff and clumsy, which makes typing a bit of a challenge. I make many more typing mistakes than I used to, often hitting more than one key at a time, or the wrong key all together. My current finger dexterity and eyesight make working on the computer a different challenge.

Then there is breathing, which doesn't surprise me. As the diaphragm muscle weakens, breathing is going to become harder and harder. Respiratory problems are what kill most people with ALS and will likely kill me. I have to say that is a little scary. If there is anything that will get me in a panic mode, it's not being able to breathe.

As ALS progresses, fatigue becomes a bigger and bigger issue. Just wheeling myself across a room in my manual wheelchair is now enough to get me winded, and I'm almost always sleepy, even though I get around twelve hours of sleep in a day.

The one thing that hasn't declined is my happiness. I'm still happy 99% of the time, and despite the progression of my ALS, in good spirits. How could I not be, when I can sit at my computer listening to Rimsky-Korsakov's Scheherazade, as our little dog lies sleeping on my feet? I'm extra glad that I have the luxury to enjoy my family, including our dog. And I'm glad my mental state isn't faltering, as the rest of my body spirals downward.

This is the latest on the progression of my progressive disease. I still hate what the ALS Monster is doing to me but refuse to give the Monster the satisfaction of making me bitter. Self-pity isn't going to make the Monster go away; it just makes him stronger. And, I'm not going to give the Monster that, while he continues to rob me.

Youthful Happiness and Optimism

14 November 2018

Yesterday afternoon I was delighted to see that my sister's granddaughter had posted a short video of the highlights of her recent wedding on Facebook. It was fun for Connie and me to watch the video and see the youthful optimism of the young couple. I loved seeing their obvious love for each other and the abundance of happiness. It made me smile inside, and I hoped that their life together will be filled with the blessings of love.

After watching the video twice, I scrolled on down the Facebook site and saw a post on one of the ALS sites that I watch. In that post I saw a young woman who is the same age as my sister's granddaughter. The young woman had just been diagnosed with ALS, and she was reaching out for support from people in her age bracket who are also facing the challenges of ALS. Reading that young woman's post and then some of her follow up comments, I could tell that she had had all her dreams crushed with the diagnosis of ALS. Like my sister's granddaughter, the young woman was recently married, and I'm sure she was looking at a bright future before her ALS diagnosis.

Over the last couple of years, I've seen several Facebook posts by young people facing ALS. They always break my heart, especially when young people have kids of their own. One young woman posts about her experience as a young mother living with ALS. Her posts almost always make me cry, but I also smile inside, because in her postings, it's obvious that her extra cute toddler is loved and cared for. Another young lady posted that her ALS symptoms started shortly after she found out that she was pregnant, and then her diagnosis came just two months before her first child was born. One woman posted that her ALS progressed so rapidly that she could not hold her baby and could only watch as others took care of her child. There is also a young father who posts from time to time. From his posts I've learned that he has to talk to his young son using eye-gaze technology and a computer-generated voice. So, anytime I'm feeling sorry for myself, I remember how lucky I've been, compared to these young people that I have little in common with, except our shared disease.

It's no secret that amyotrophic lateral sclerosis (ALS) is a seriously devastating disease. There is no cure, and the one given is that the disease will continue to progress. The biggest unknown is the rate of the decline. The statistics say that life expectancy is three to five years. That stat doesn't leave a lot of room to be optimistic. But, like all statistics, there are exceptions to the rule. I frequently read posts on Facebook by people who have been living with ALS for over ten years, some even twenty. Don't forget, Stephen Hawking lived over fifty years with ALS, and that was after he was told upon diagnosis that he'd likely live only two years. Sadly, the rate that ALS runs its course seems to be faster in young people than in people in my age bracket. One young lady, a mother of a toddler, was posting just about a year ago, how she had just been diagnosed. In that time, she has lost her ability to walk, is losing her ability to talk, now gets her nourishment via a feed tube and will soon need a tracheotomy ventilator. All in less than a year.

As sad as it is reading the posts of these young people, sadder yet was reading about a young boy who is ten and has familial ALS that was passed down to him by his mother. The article said that, in the US, he is one of just four kids younger than a teenager with ALS. And his symptoms started presenting at age four. It is extra sad that children have their youth robbed from them by such a terrible disease.

As much as I hate having ALS, I know that I have lived a happy adult life with my wonderful wife. We might have struggled a few times to make ends meet, but we never were hungry, lacked shelter, or lived in a land that was devastated by war. So I feel lucky. Especially when I consider the young people that I have mentioned. I watched my son mature into a man with his own family, and I've been lucky enough to have three grandsons. In spite of ALS, I hope the young parents that I have mentioned get to see their children grow up. I also hope that they are lucky enough to feel the magic of being a grandparent.

Doctor Letters

21 November 2018

Since I can't talk, I always write a letter to the doctor I'm about to visit. Below is a letter I wrote to my primary care doctor, Dr. Hunter. I don't know if records get transferred to Dr. Hunter, so I like to keep him up to date on my medical visits to Seattle. I'm extra lucky to have such a good and dedicated doctor as I do in Dr. Hunter. He is the best.

To:	*Dr. Hunter*
Date:	*November 21, 2018*
Regarding:	*Marcel LaPerriere*

Virginia Mason Visits

1. In September I saw Dr. Govier, a Urologist, at Virginia Mason. He did a scope of my bladder and did a digital exam of my prostate. He found the bladder looked okay. The prostate was a bit enlarged, but he didn't feel any abnormal growths. Here are his exact words regarding my elevated PAS: "If you had 10 to 15 more years to live, we would look for cancer. In your case, you're much more likely to die from ALS, than prostate cancer."

2. I did have a bladder infection, but the antibiotics that you prescribed in August did the trick. However, Dr. Govier wanted to recheck my urine in October.

3. I went back to Virginia Mason in late October and saw Dr. Porter. No further infection was found. Both Dr. Porter and Dr. Govier felt that my prostate might have caused the infection. Dr. Porter agreed with Dr. Govier, and both see no reason to ever test my PSA in the future.

4. Dr. Porter said to say hi to you. When Connie asked him, if he knew you, this is what he said, "Yes, I know him well. He is a very good doctor and a nice guy." We concur.

5. In October I saw Virginia Mason endocrinologist, Dr. Stoehr, about my high FSH and low testosterone, as well as hormones associated with Acromegaly. He feels that supplementing testosterone would do more harm than good, especially considering the potential of prostate cancer. He said that could accelerate the growth of abnormal cells.

6. Dr. Stoehr also sees no reason to check growth hormones or IGF1 in the future since both were normal three years post-surgery.

What's New

1. I quit the Breo Ellipta. I no longer have the inhalation strength to inhale it into my lungs. When I'd accidentally forget to take it, I didn't see any difference. Is there a pill that could do something like the Ellipta?

2. Two or three days after stopping the Breo, I did notice what I assume was withdrawal symptoms, because they were symptoms like I've had when I stopped other steroids too quickly.

3. I think I will soon need the settings increased on my BIPAP. Currently, the inspiratory pressure is 10 and the expiratory pressure is 5. Geneva Woods can do that remotely. We didn't see a pulmonologist in Seattle, so I'm not sure what we need to do. You mentioned an allergist come to Sitka. Is that something he could do?

4. Might need a portable BIPAP soon; something that I can use during the day when I'm up and about. Again, I wonder if this is something that the allergist can prescribe?

5. Should I see Mr. Hanson the pulmonary therapist at SEARHC?

6. On our two-month-long road trip, I had to use the prednisone you prescribed. I had a bad attack in Wyoming. I find the prednisone helps greatly. In fact, I had some left over from a long time ago and found that 5 mg works well as a maintenance dosage. I know we have talked about this before, but I wonder if I should just stay on 5 mg? I know the cons of doing that. So, it's hard to weigh the pros and cons.

7. Other declines are my eyelids are not opening all the way, which messes with my vision. Also, my fingers are declining. Especially on my left. That means shorter notes to you from me in the future.

Have a great Thanksgiving.

Marcel LaPerriere

Postscript: Dr. Hunter did give me a prescription for a daily dosage of 5 mg of Pred-nisone, which has helped with my breathing. Also, I got my BIPAP machine turned up to 12 on the inspiratory pressure and seven on the expiratory pressure. I'm still waiting for a portable unit. If all goes well, I'll get one mid-April.

Fasciculations

29 November 2018

Everyone from time to time gets a muscle spasm or twitching. But people with ALS have many more than those who don't. In my case, the twitching, or fasciculations as they are called in the medical world, are nearly daily and sometimes nonstop. The other thing about fasciculations –– at least in my case and for most people with ALS –– they are a precursor to further decline. Lately my left thumb has been twitching. I had already been noticing the decline of mobility in my fingers, but lately, the decline seems to be speeding up, especially in my left hand. That totally scares me, because my hands are the way I communicate. I never appreciated how important one's hands are. Just this morning I was noting how much harder it is to get dressed when my left hand refused to function properly. And little things –– like grabbing a spoon from the flatware drawer, opening and closing a Ziploc bag, turning a page in the newspaper or grabbing a single pill out of a prescription bottle –– are getting to be a real challenge.

Because I depend on my hands to communicate, I was glad Connie and I had a Facetime conversation with the Assistive Technology Professional at the Evergreen Chapter of the ALS Association. She explored with us the technologies out there if I get to a point that I can no longer use my hands to type what I want to say. It's comforting to know that the Evergreen Chapter of the ALS Association is there to help.

But needing help communicating might be a moot point because my breathing is failing. It now seems to be a race between the failure in my ability to breathe and the failure of my fingers. It's already very hard to blow my nose, and when I attempt coughing, I'm only successful about 20% of the time. A simple head or chest cold, or worse, a combination, could be fatal. I won't live in an isolation bubble out of fear of catching a cold. I just take as many precautions as possible, keeping my hands clean, getting lots of rest and eating as healthily as I can.

Though I have a cough assist machine, I don't seem to be able to get used to it. In fact, I hate it with a passion. The blasted thing blows air into my lungs, then sucks it back out. It also seems to blow air into my stomach, and then sucks that back out too. So, every time I use it, no matter how I have my neck positioned, I either vomit of come close to vomiting. When I asked for suggestions on one of the ALS Facebook sites, others said they have no problems, and one lady said her husband loves his. So maybe it's just me.

Back to fasciculations. My left eyelid is twitching as well. If I don't get plenty of sleep –– this means in excess of eleven hours in twenty-four –– I can't open my eyes enough to see clearly. This, too, is concerning. Three years ago, it was bad enough to lose my ability to talk. Now the thought of losing my eyesight is one more thing to fear.

It's a given that ALS sucks. But I'm not going to give in to the ALS Monster and be bitter over the things it is stealing from me. Daily I enjoy my family, our daily walks –– which in my case means a power wheelchair ride. And our little beagle, Bella, makes me smile each day. In spite of ALS, my life is full of too many blessings to count. Life is good.

Money

4 December 2018

When a devastating disease hits, the last thing one wants to worry about is its financial burden on the family. But everyone who is hit with a disease like ALS, cancer, or even a bad injury, must face the reality that getting sick is expensive. My wife and I are very lucky in that regard. I'm not happy that we have had to use our savings for my illness instead of the travel we had planned. But at least we had some savings, and we both have pensions. Others are not always that lucky.

A couple of young people that I follow on Facebook are like most of us when we were young –– we expected everything to go smoothly, with a mortgage and car payments. In an instant everything changes when the devastating news of ALS slaps them and their family in the face. Not only do they have to spend money on things that they never thought they'd have to, like home modifications or a different automobile to transport them and their power-wheelchair, but as the disease progresses, they can no longer work. One woman created a Go Fund Me page, something I know she didn't want to do. The last I looked she is only 1/6th of the way to her goal with diminishing hope that she will raise the money that she needs to modify her house. Another disabled woman living on a fixed income must suddenly have her young adult son with ALS move in with her so she can be his caregiver.

My union pension from the City of Ketchikan is not large, but it pays our mortgage. And our two Social Security pensions pay our daily expenses and other bills. We had to dig into our savings for medical travel and the handicap van we purchased. Little did I know, when I'd stick money into a 401K, that instead of using it for something fun in our retirement, we'd have to spend it for things that are not so fun. Because we live in a small, remote Alaska town, we must travel to Seattle for anything major dealing with my ALS. I've long ago lost track of how many medical-related trips we have made to Seattle in the last four years, but it must be around twenty. Each trip, when you add up airfare and hotels, costs an average of well over $2,000.00 –– a big chip from our savings each time we are forced to go south. Insurance, Medicare and my Medigap insurance don't cover all medical expenses.

Our house was mostly already set up for my progressing immobility because we built it with Connie's elderly mother living with us in mind. All the ramps were already in place, as well as a mostly handicapped accessible bathroom. Either I, or my grandson Blake under my direction, made the additional modifications that were needed, which saved us a ton of money that others must spend in order to continue to live in their own homes.

Financially it would make the most sense to move to the continental United States to be closer to larger, better equipped medical facilities, but we love living where we do. ALS has robbed so much from us that we don't want where we live taken from us, too. Yesterday morning, on our daily walk, we had a long talk about the quality of life with a very nice man who works in the local medical field. He, too, thinks that living where we want to live plays an important part in the life quality we seek. I was grateful he took the time for our visit because it helped me more clearly see there are more important things than extending life as long as you can. It costs more and will continue to cost us more to live where we do, but it's worth it.

The number one reason for personal bankruptcy in the USA is due to unexpected medical expenses. I'm glad that we likely will not have to face that, and I feel for others who do. Imagine, already facing the challenges of dealing with a major medical issue, plus the financial ramifications of that illness. That is heartbreaking, especially when it's a widow or widower who has lost their loved one. We are lucky that ALS didn't strike until we had accumulated some financial security with savings and pensions. We are not doing what we had wanted to do in our retirement years, but we both know things could be much worse.

I would love to wave some magic wand and help many others dealing with the financial strains associated with medical care, and I did donate to the woman's Go Fund Me page. But Connie and I must be prudent with our own hard-earned money and "save it for a rainy day." Several people have said I was unlucky to get ALS, but I often feel like I'm the luckiest guy in the world. We are far from rich, but we have enough money to feel financially secure. I have the best family ever, and I live in a beautiful location. I'm darned lucky.

Why Is Love So Hard to Say?

5 December 2018

It's hard for me to say, "I love you, too." I'm, of course, speaking metaphorically, because I can't physically speak at all. When family or friends respond to one of my Facebook posts, with an "I love you," or when we are on the phone, and someone in my family says the same, I truly wish I could respond, "I love you." It's not that I don't want to, but to do so, I pick open psychological scars, that knowing what I now know, might be a mild case of post-traumatic stress syndrome. Without a professional diagnosis I'll never know, but even when I could talk, it was nearly impossible for me to say those words. Just like it was always very hard for me to hug anyone but my wife.

I've only told Connie, my son when he was little, and my grandsons when they were little, I loved them. I may have said "I love you" when I was younger than seven, before my mother died, but I don't remember. When my father remarried less than a year after the death of our mother, my two sisters and I lived in a totally dysfunctional hell house that had no love within its walls. I often heard "I love you," but those words were as false as if I were to say, "Potatoes grow on trees." When my dad or stepmother said anything to do with love, there was no truth in it. An "I love you," spoken in public by my dad or stepmother, was often followed by a beating once out of the public eye.

I read a few years ago about a woman who had sadly experienced a brutal rape. Years after her rape, she would walk into a safe location like a bank or a grocery store and she would start panicking. She had no idea why this panic overcame her, and her only relief was to escape as fast as she could. Over time and with therapy, she discovered the triggering mechanism for her was the smell of a popular men's deodorant. The rapist must have been wearing that same fragrance when he raped her. Every time she'd encounter that smell, it would trigger something deep in her brain and she'd understandably panic. Once she understood what was causing her anxiety, she was better able to handle it, but not eliminate it.

Unlike the rape victim, sometimes a panic mechanism is more obvious. When I was in high school working in a small machine shop across the street from where I was living, one of my fellow employees was a young man who had recently returned from Vietnam, where he had seen combat. One day, while running a metal lathe, he didn't properly engage the gears when he changed the lathe into what is called "back gear." Since the gears were not properly engaged when he turned on the lathe, there was the sound of, "rat a tat tat, rat a tat tat," exploding for a few seconds until it jumped totally out of gear. Standing at our own lathes, we laughed as the man jumped to the floor and placed his hands over his head. A few seconds later as he stood up trembling like a leaf and obviously very shaken, we saw that it was no laughing matter. The subconscious can be much more powerful than the conscious mind. His actions switched the machine on and caused the sound of a machine gun to emanate from within. Yet he had no control over what his body did. He was so dazed by the experience that one of the bosses had to take him home.

More than fifty years have passed since I lived under my parent's roof, but I still occasionally have nightmares from the beatings. I also carry some deep scars that have not totally healed. At one time, when someone other than Connie would go to hug me, I'd want to run and cower in a corner with my hands over my head. Sometimes, I used to even feel physically sick when someone would try to hug me, or for sure if they said, "I love you." It has taken me the better part of forty years to get over wanting to run and hide. Those wounds are what give me the inability to return an "I love you" when a family member says it to me. I wish I could get over it, especially now that I have ALS, and know that family members are expressing their deep concern by saying those three little words, "I love you."

One of the things I miss the most about not being able to talk is saying "I love you" to Connie. For over forty years, "I love you" was how each day would start and end. I greatly miss that. That is possibly the most painful thing about not being able to talk.

If the woman who was raped, the young man who was running the machine tool, and I stood next to each other, on the surface it would look like we have nothing in common. All three of us have deep-seated mental wounds that partially control who we are. Sometimes, there are things beyond our control that shape us. We might want our personalities to be different, but as hard as we try to change them, we can't. During my whole adult life I would have liked to be more open with affection towards the people I care about than I ever was.

The worst is abusing children. Not only do the mental scars run deep, but who knows what physical maladies will result down the line from the abuse. Anecdotally, there is very strong evidence that head trauma can cause ALS and other neurology disorders. When you look at football players from around the world, both American football and what we call soccer, there is a much higher propensity for ALS in those people than in the general population. Just recently I learned that ALS is more common in National Hockey League Players than the population at large. And, might the fact that military veterans also have a higher ratio of ALS than civilians, also be related to head trauma? The brain is a very complex and sensitive organ that needs protection from both physical and mental abuse -- especially during childhood.

Back to those three little words, "I love you." I apologize to my family and friends that I find those words so hard to say in writing and physically, when I could still talk. I do very much appreciate that you care enough for me to say them, and please understand why it so hard for me. It took me the better part of four decades to get over my hatred of receiving hugs. Now, if I only had a bit more time to get over my fear of those three little words.

Hands

9 December 2018

I usually listen to classical music while typing these essays. Ever since I was a kid, I've loved the music of Bach, Mozart, Beethoven, or my favorite, Brahms, and so many more. If I'm not listening to instrumental music, I listen to opera, or lately, choral music. I'm not sure why it took me so long to appreciate the beauty of good choral music, but now that I've found it, I'm hooked.

What does music have to do with "Hands," the title of this essay? All the music we love, no matter what genre, requires hands, and in most cases, the composer had to write it down. What separates us from other animals, besides our brain, is our hands with opposing thumbs. All the classical instruments would be darn hard to play without an opposing thumb. And how could any classical master composer have written down his magical music without functioning hands?

Choral music, my new musical discovery, is performed in some of the most beautiful cathedrals of the world. Though I've never personally heard one of the requiems I love so much sung in a cathedral, I've visited many of "Europe's amazingly beautiful cathedrals. One, the Duomo in Milan, Italy, took over 400 years to build. Imagine how many people and how many pairs of hands built such a masterpiece.

Connie and I have also been lucky enough to see the artworks of da Vinci, Michelangelo, Donatello, Rembrandt, Vincent van Gogh, and many others. The paintings of those brilliantly talented men would not have been possible without hands. Standing in front of da Vinci's painting, "The Last Supper," brings tears to your eyes, and it's humbling to walk through the Louvre in Paris with amazing statues and paintings everywhere you look.

It's not only our brains that give us a little immortality, but our hands. The men that laid the foundation for the Milan Duomo did it over 600 years ago with no idea what the completed building would look like. Because of their craftsmanship, the building still stands as a tribute to all who helped build it. Though Bach has been dead for almost 270 years, his work lives on and will likely live on for the rest of humanity. That's immortality. Nothing my hands ever created will live on like that, but I still take pride in the fact that many things I made will live on past my death.

Other than our brains and our face, nothing defines who we are more than our hands. That's why losing the ability to maneuver my hands scares me so much. Not only do I depend on my hands to type what I want to say, but how long will I still able to feed and bathe myself? If I lose hand mobility before I die, that means I'll depend on others for the things that will keep me alive. That is the extra frightening thing, because I don't want to depend on others -- especially knowing what a burden that will be for Connie.

A woman I've mentioned before said the most painful thing was losing the ability to brush her own hair when she lost the use of her arms and hands. Feeding herself, bathing herself, or even being able to wipe after using the toilet would have been more painful to me. But our hair is our public face. It tells others much about who we are. How she created her daily hair design with her hands might have been the one creative thing she did each day to satisfy that human need.

With over 3000 sensory nerve receptors in each finger, no part of our body is more important to express love than our hands are. We kiss with our lips, but the tender touch of a hand expresses love much more than a kiss. I've told Connie how much I love her by holding hands or tenderly patting part of her body. The first time I held my newborn son while holding the hand of my wife created a true bond of love that would have been hard without hands. Nothing can compare with the feeling of holding your grandchild in your hands for the first time. The most satisfying thing was when one of my grandsons would reach up to grab my hands. Each time one of my grandsons would hold my hand to cross a street, my heart melted.

As I sit here typing with my hands, I'm listening to "Scheherazade," one of the most beautiful pieces of music ever written, composed by the hands of Rimsky-Korsakov. Looking at my hands as they type each letter, I'm proud of all the things I made in hopes of making life better for others. In my machinist/tool and diemaker days, my hands made everything: parts that helped the space program, surgical instruments, plastic injection and blow molds for the food container industry, parts for many airplanes, and too many others to list. I'm proud of the power generation equipment that these hands put together or maintained and of the houses I helped build. And I'm proud these hands typed, or hand wrote more letters to government officials and politicians that I can count. If even one of those letters helped, I can rest in peace knowing that my hands contributed to the world I live in. ALS is causing my hands and body to waste away, but ALS can never take away the things I've accomplished with my hands. I'll never have even a small bit of immortality the masters I've mentioned have, but I have created many things that will live well past my death. And that brings me joy.

Phone

11 December 2018

With the exception of texting, I don't use my smartphone as a phone. Instead, it's my main way of communicating and many other things like reading the news, listening to podcasts, taking photos, navigating via GPS, and, when traveling, as a tool to find places to take our dog, Bella, for a walk. Since I can't talk, I can't answer the phone when it does ring. I let it go to voice mail and if it is an important call, I ask Connie to call back.

Because I use the same phone number I have had for years, and the number was once listed as my business number, I still get calls associated with my long-ago shuttered business. Most of those calls are solicitors looking to sell something, or, in some cases, all-out fraud. A recent message said, "Hi —— this is John, and I have ten jobs lined up in your neighborhood, and I need a contractor to help me get the projects knocked out." When I look at the number, it was from Tampa, Florida. The realistic chances that John has ten jobs lined up in the small Alaska town that I live in? Zero. So, I block calls from numbers like that.

If I get two calls from the same number with no message, I block it. Over the last couple of years, I kept getting calls from various numbers in Holly, Colorado. Even after blocking, yesterday when I received yet another call from that location, I decided to answer it. "Gerrrr... ummmmm... gerrr... burrrr," I groaned into my iPhone. I heard a woman on the other end, and I then hung up. It's not polite to hang up, so I quickly called back and got the message, "Hello this is Melisa, I'm away from my phone right now, so please leave a message and I'll call you right back." I left this message, "Gerrrr... ummmmm... gerrr... burrrr," then asked Connie to call back and tell them to take me off their list, which she did in a slightly angry voice, explaining that I can't talk because of ALS.

Not knowing where Holly, Colorado is, I decided to Google it. It's a small town east of Pueblo, on the Kansas border. Since it is a small town, I must assume that all the numbers I've blocked from there over the last couple of years were likely all from the same company. Each time I'd block one of their numbers, they'd just call back on a different number. I don't feel at all guilty about my, " Gerrrr... ummmmm... gerrr... burrrrr," and in fact, if I ever get another call that says it's from there, they will get the same or a variation of the same.

When I was still able to talk, I hated calls from telemarketers trying to sell me something, especially if they interrupted something important. One company, Capital Contractors, became so obnoxious I reported them repeatedly to the Federal Communications Commission (FCC). I'm not sure the FCC did anything, though the Capital Contractors callers often resorted to the most-foul language you can imagine when I'd say I wasn't interested. Then they started calling my home number and Connie had to face their extra foul behavior.

Now that I've been out of business for over two years, I still get texts, trying to sell me things –– usually a business loan or a business credit card. I've been politely texting back, asking them to take me off their list, which doesn't always work. Maybe it's time to have some fun there too? Next time I'll text back something like this, "Oh, thank goodness, you're my salvation! I need a million dollars ASAP. Can you PLEASE HELP? If I don't get that money by next Monday, Guido says he is going to give me some concrete overshoes and drop me in the harbor." Or should I just text back, " Gerrrr... ummmmm... gerrr... burrrrr?" A guy has gotta have a little fun.

Love and Empathy

14 December 2018

Most mornings, as I roll around the kitchen in my wheelchair making my breakfast, I listen to the New York Times podcast, The Daily, hosted by Michael Barbaro. The usual format is Mr. Barbaro doing an in-depth interview with New York Times reporters about one of the more pertinent news stories of the day. A few days ago, Mr. Barbaro was interviewing photojournalist Tyler Hicks about his haunting photo of a starving Yemani seven-year-old girl that has been published world-wide. Mr. Hicks told how he came about taking the photo, followed by the sad story of how the girl died two weeks after the photo was taken. The story then, and now, brings tears to my eyes. How sad and terrible the little girl's death must have been for her parents. It's stories like that, that make me realize that I have no right to ever feel sorry for myself. I have a fatal disease that is wasting my body away, but I'm 100% luckier than the poor father who, out of no fault of his own, had to watch his daughter die of starvation.

Abraham Lincoln supposedly said that empathy is the most important personal attribute. I'd add to say if we humans were more empathetic, the world would be a better place. Would we engage in wars if we felt empathy for those we call our enemies? If politicians were more empathetic, wouldn't they find solutions that would help all the people they are elected to represent? What about the world's wealthiest 1%, who now hold around half of the world's wealth? If they had more empathy, wouldn't they share some of their wealth with the less fortunate?

I have a long way to go to become empathetic. However, one of the strange side effects of ALS might be empathy. Emotions become more heightened in many people with ALS. Some people have spontaneous laughter and others have bouts of crying. I'm now much more sensitive to emotional stories like the one above. Nowadays it's hard for me to get through the daily news without coming close to

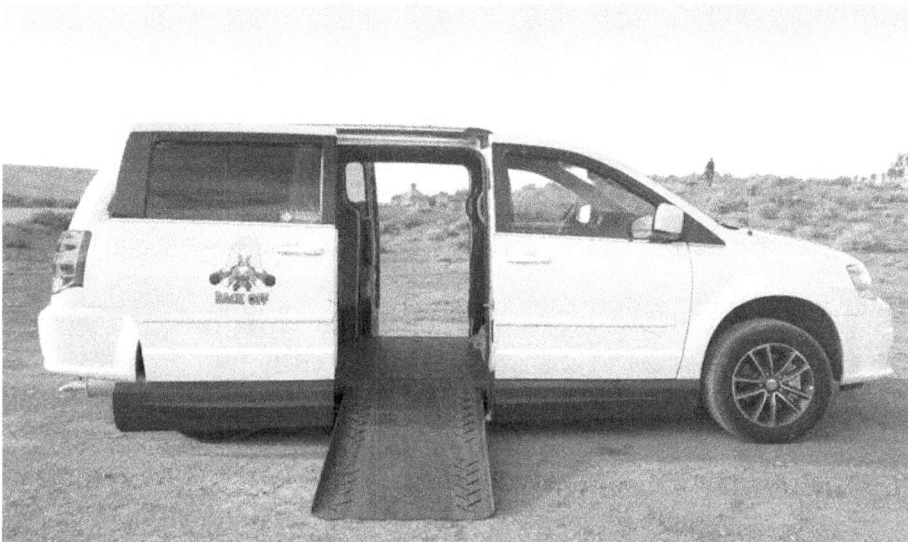

September 2018. Our van in Utah.

crying or with a tear or two running down my cheek. I also can't look at the videos that pop up on Facebook of animal cruelty without crying. Isn't sadness also sometimes empathy? In my case it is.

The other day, shortly after I lay down for a nap, my son, Zach walked in the back door and yelled, "Howdy." Since I can't answer, I moved to my wheelchair, rolled into the living room, and heard Zach say, "I can tell when you're home by the squeaky bed. That would drive me crazy, but I guess you're used to it." It does drive me a little crazy and, yes, I'm used to it. But I'm darn lucky to have the hospital-type bed that Medicare and my insurance paid for.

It might be squeaky, but it makes life easier for me and more comfortable than a regular bed. Others with ALS aren't even lucky enough to have a bed. I've watched a video of a poor ALS sufferer around my age who, living in the mountains in India, has neither a bed nor a wheelchair. His adult sons lift him from a pad on the floor to a chair, and if he wants to go outside for some sun, they carry him out to a bench with his back to the wall. Knowing how hard it is to breathe while sleeping lying flat without a BIPAP ventilator, I can't imagine how he gets along. I depend on that $4500.00 machine to breathe when I sleep, but even if he had a BIPAP machine, he wouldn't have the power to operate it. I'm not going to complain about a few squeaks when I have both a bed and a machine that makes sleep easier for me.

You don't have to go all the way to India to see how much more fortunate I am than others with ALS. In another video, a young woman demonstrated how she feeds herself via her PEG feeding tube. When she had the PEG surgically implanted, she had to ride the bus to the hospital and then home again by herself. She is not the only person who is facing ALS without the help and support of loved ones. I'm so amazingly lucky to have my wonderful wife, Connie, helping me along the path of ALS, and I feel for anyone who has to face ALS without a supportive family.

We are also lucky to have our own handicapped equipped van. Part of keeping a good mental attitude is the ability to get outside and take in some fresh air. The van lets me get to places in our small town that I could never get to without it. I'm lucky and I feel for others facing ALS without an easy way of getting out of their houses.

Because we have ALS in common, it's easy for me to have empathy for the man in India, and even the young woman in the feeding tube video. It's even easy for me to have empathy for the man in Yemen who lost his daughter to starvation, even though our only common ground is that we are both fathers. I sometimes struggle with having empathy for people who have a different political view than I do. Twenty-years ago, a man thirty years my senior told me, "Always assume that your adversaries are good people and have good intentions. If you don't agree with them, that's okay, but do your best to respect them." Those wise words could help lead all of us to live a more empathetic life.

Volunteering

21 December 2018

I find it almost unbelievable when someone says they have no regrets, as I have a ton of them. I regret that I didn't spend more time with my family; that way too often I put work ahead of family time and play; that I didn't travel more. And, crazy as it might sound, I regret not volunteering more time.

We hoped to spend our retirement years traveling and volunteering. I fantasized a cross-country road trip, stopping to volunteer with organizations like Habitat for Humanity, working on a trail in one of America's many wilderness areas, or helping clean up after a hurricane or some other natural disaster.

The greatest and often the most rewarding work I've done as an adult has been volunteer work. I served on several nonprofit boards, but most rewarding was more tangible work –– work where I'd get my hands dirty. Over the last 15 years I've volunteered a full year with the US Forest Service, doing everything from caving to helping build a log cabin. Though often frustrated by the bureaucracy of the USFS, I kept going back because the work was darn fun. I was also making a tiny contribution to one of America's treasures, our public lands. And USFS volunteering involved travel to places that I wouldn't have had a chance to visit otherwise.

The best people I've ever known are people who give of themselves –– volunteers. At Sheldon Jackson College (SJC) my job was overseeing and working with some 1000 volunteers, on whom SJC survival and day to day operations depended. SJC was loosely tied to the Presbyterian Church and their nation-wide volunteer recruitment resource. That the campus was located in Alaska didn't hurt attracting volunteers.

Little did I know when we moved to Sitka in 2003 that I'd end up with the toughest, but most rewarding, job of my adult life. A few days before Christmas, just as the college went on the holiday break, I started work at SJC as the Maintenance Director. Before I applied for the job, a campus walking tour showed that years of deferred maintenance had left the buildings in poor shape. And if the outside of the buildings looked that rough, things would be just as bad or worse inside. I soon learned the main campus buildings were fewer than a third of the buildings that I'd be responsible for maintaining. I'd also be overseeing four full-time and three part-time janitors, and for some crazy reason, the one full-time night-time security guard. My staff for this: one volunteer and one student. That's over 40 buildings to maintain with one volunteer, one-part time student and myself. I was crazy to take the job and maybe crazier to stay. I'm glad I did stick it out because of all the wonderful people I had the privilege of meeting and a darn good boss.

My first day I was introduced to my first Volunteer in Mission (VIM), Chuck, a retired minister and the one volunteer on the maintenance team. Before he and his wife, Jan, left for two weeks in Portland, OR, he showed me what I and my part-time student helper needed to do during Christmas break. As Chuck took me in one building after another, showing me the boiler rooms and so many other things that would need attention, I gained real respect for this man who had been thrust into an impossible job that he didn't expect when he signed up to be a VIM. When Chuck and Jan started their year-long commitment at SJC, there was a Maintenance Director. That man quit after four months, and Chuck suddenly found himself the Acting Director of Maintenance. That he didn't leave, even though the stress caused him to have a significant flair-up of the shingles, impressed me significantly. Chuck was my first lesson on how dedicated volunteers can be. I still find it amazing that he took on the job and stuck it out for over two months until I was hired.

The two-week Christmas break went by quickly because I was so busy with things breaking down that I hardly had time to go home. Sitka experienced a major freezing spell during that time, and not only did many pipes freeze, but several heating systems broke down. I was delighted to see Chuck return because I could turn over the less demanding jobs to him. Chuck and I made a good team and I was very happy he signed up for another year.

About the first week in February, Charley, the first of many short-term VIM's, showed up for a two-week work stint. I was immediately impressed by how much an additional volunteer could help keep my head above water. Soon Charley was crawling around in attics of the main dorm building, helping me remove three HVAC heat exchanger coils that had frozen. And, when all the ovens in the cafeteria failed, it was Charley who helped me troubleshoot the electrical wiring problem that had shorted them out. I was sure sad when Charley's two weeks ended.

Fortunately, Dale, a retired carpenter from North Dakota, showed up for a three-month stay. He didn't have the overall skills Charley had, but he was a darn good carpenter who could repair broken doors and windows as well as a thousand other tasks.

And Chuck continued to be worth his weight in gold by taking over the majority of the ordering and paperwork. He was also the campus locksmith and cared for the thousands of locks that always needed to be fixed or changed.

By March I was starting to see the value that other VIMs brought to the campus. There were VIMs working in the library, teaching classes, operating the cash register in the cafeteria, working the main desk in the gym, and manning most of the offices required to keep a college operational. It was also in March when I learned about workgroups.

A meeting held in the president's office building included the president's assistant, Ann, the volunteer coordinator (my boss) Fred, and myself. I was asked what my plans were for the summer workgroups. I asked, "What are workgroups?" Each summer about a dozen to fifteen churches each sent from 10 to 20 volunteers to work in maintenance, and these groups usually came to Sitka for two weeks. My job was not only to oversee their work but to come up with projects for them. It was a good thing I was sitting down. I had known that a few volunteers would come to work on the grounds, mowing lawns and taking care of flower beds, but I had no idea that up to 200 plus people would come each summer and that they'd fall under my direction. It scared me to death. After the meeting, I met separately with Fred. He, too, was relatively new to his position. I'm not sure he knew much more about workgroups than I did. He had observed a couple of workgroups the previous summer from his office window, and it looked like someone was trying to herd cats -- they all looked lost without anyone leading them. Besides the impossibility of maintaining buildings, many around 100 years old, I began to understand why my predecessor only lasted a few months.

I was writing my resignation letter in my head as I walked across the campus to my office. My job was nearly impossible as it was, with way too much work to do, almost no money to do the work, no skilled workforce and endless breakdowns. How was I going to oversee a steady stream of volunteers?

At Fred's request, I wrote up a list of projects that needed to be done on campus, put a priority on each, and calculated the cost of materials for each.

Marcel LaPerriere

The list was nearly twenty pages long. I asked people with minimal mechanical or carpenter skills willing to work under my direction to put a dent in the years and years of deferred maintenance. And this is going to sound crazy. I started getting excited.

The 2003/04 school year soon came to an end, and my first work-groups started showing up. One of the first groups was from Rochester, MN, and around half of the twenty-some people worked at the Mayo Clinic. Several were doctors, including the head eye surgeon and his wife. They also had a man who owned a landscaping and handyman business, so I had at least one partially skilled worker. And they brought money to finance the projects I had reserved for them. Their main project was replacing the leaking roof on the Maintenance Building. Though I took some grief from the president of the College for not focusing on the more visible buildings, I could easily justify the project –– without a building to work from, how could we do maintenance? Thanks to a record-breaking nice summer, we not only got the roof replaced but accomplished much of the work that I had on my list.

Also that summer, a surprise caller asked if I could keep 80 teenaged kids busy for the week that they'd be on campus. Wow, a surprise group of 80 teens all the way from Pennsylvania. On top of two other full workgroups, I'd now have 80 kids to find work for and supervise. The local Presbyterian Church housed the kids but could find work for 20 of them. That left me 60 teenagers and around 40 adults from the other two workgroups to supervise that week.

The kids were great. I soon had several of them with hand tools brushing along side the flume that was still being used to supply water to the fish hatchery. About 20 girls adopted one of the dirtiest and most physically challenging job I ever asked any volunteers to do. An 8500 sq. footprint classroom building had just undergone a complete remodel of the interior. Before my time, past workgroups and the contractor who did the remodel tossed tons and tons of rotted wood, rusted pipes, old wire and lots of other stuff into the crawlspace when the floor was opened to replace rotted floor joists. The crawlspace in that building was a lake of mud –– in some places, the mud and water were over two feet deep. Though I gave the girls rubber boots, rain gear, and duct-tape to tape their rain gear to the boots, they still got totally covered in mud. Every time I'd stick my head through the crawlspace door, I'd see a long line of hunched-over giggling girls passing crud, oozing with mud in bucket-brigade fashion. I would have loved to have submitted a few photos of those girls, with mud dripping on their faces, in their hair and all over their rain gear and clothing, to a teen fashion magazine. They did a fantastic job, and I loved watching them rib the boys who were too squeamish to take on the job of mucking in the mud.

After my first summer of overseeing workgroups, I couldn't wait for the next summer. It was a lot of work, but also a lot of fun. The best thing was all the wonderful people I met.

Due to years of poor management, the college closed its doors in 2007, and over one hundred employees lost their jobs. I still feel bitter about the closure. I enjoyed the students and the staff that worked at the school, but I have a special place in my heart for all the volunteers.

As I was finishing this up, I received a Christmas card from a woman who came two different summers to be part of a workgroup. That card made my day, especially knowing that this lady, who lives on the east coast, is a top management executive working in one of the largest accounting firms in the world. She thanked me for giving her confidence in herself and for giving her good lasting memories. All I did was ask her to lay vinyl tile in one of the family housing apartments, something she had never done. She and her fellow volunteers were reluctant to take on the task, and after a little arm twisting and a little training, they did a great job. They may not have been as fast as a pro, but they did every bit as good as a pro would have.

Marcel LaPerriere

I regret that ALS robbed me of the volunteer work I had hoped to do. It can never steal from me all the good memories and friends I made at Sheldon Jackson College. Many of those past volunteers are now my Facebook friends -- to list all their names would take most of a page. I hope they all know what a privilege it was for me to work with them and now call them friends. All are cream of the crop when it comes to good people. I am honored to have spent time with them.

Time and Energy

26 December 2018

I could also add productivity to the title because ALS robs all three from its victims. As ALS advances, fatigue and the lack of energy become more and more of a reality, at least my reality. It takes a lot more time to do the simplest things. Little things like putting on my socks now take five minutes or more, and, as crazy as it sounds, taking off my socks is just as grueling, not to mention all the things that are now almost impossible, like stairs. I could likely get up one story of stairs if I sat on my butt and scooted, but I'd shot for sure, and it would take a very long time for the round trip.

A dozen years ago when I was the Maintenance Director at Sheldon Jackson College, my day started at 4:30 am. I'd get up, quickly dress, step off our live-aboard sailboat, walk five minutes on the dock to my truck, drive five more minutes to Market Center, and still usually get to the store five minutes before it opened at 5:00 am. Louise, the morning market clerk, would open early so we half-dozen early risers could get our coffee and head off to work. Driving from Market Center to the campus took but four minutes, so I'd frequently be in my office at 5:00 am. Getting to work three hours before everyone else gave me time to get paperwork done or make progress on some projects without a ton of interruptions. This plan only backfired once, when I decided it was a good time to solder some copper pipes down in the mechanical room of the main dorm on campus. I got a little overzealous with my task, and the smoke from soldering set off the fire alarm. As I ran up the stairs to shut off the alarm, I called the fire department to let them know it was a false alarm. This made them happy, but a fire alarm in the main dorm a few minutes after 5:00 am sure didn't make the groggy-eyed students happy.

If I was lucky, my day at Sheldon Jackson ended at 6:00 pm, but I averaged about two after-hours calls a week. When I'd get called at 2:00 am for an hour or two to fix something, I'd just take a short nap in my office and work until 6:00 pm. Many times emergencies kept me on campus for one or more days. Once it was over three days when the controls for a boiler broke down, and I had to manually run it until the replacement controller made it to Sitka. I survived on a few short catnaps that I was able to grab on my office couch. Keith, the dorm RA, would spell me during those naps, or else I don't know how I would have made it.

As the first symptoms of ALS hit me, I was finishing up the last house my construction company built. Since the house was on a remote island with no road access, things like construction forklifts or a crane were luxury aids we didn't have. We had to hand move and lift everything to build that house. Every bag of concrete, every stick of wood and everything to furnish the large home had to be handled several times. I prided myself on being able to outwork all the guys who worked for me. Some of those men were 1/3 my age. I not only would work just as hard or harder, but I also always put in more hours each day and each week than they did.

Nowadays I feel like I've accomplished something if I don't have to take a nap between breakfast and lunch. And it would be nearly impossible for me to make it without an afternoon nap. Even then, I almost always feel tired. I usually average ten hours of sleep every night, and with a nap or two I average around twelve hours of sleep in twenty-four. Yesterday I outdid myself when my BIPAP machine said I slept 13.2 hours in the last twenty-four. I call my BI-PAP "Big Brother," because it tracks how much I sleep I get, reports that to the medical supply company, which in turn reports it to my pulmonologist and primary care doctors. If I don't use it at least five hours a day, it will report me to the government, meaning Medicare. Medicare requires that I use the BIPAP at least five hours in a day, or it will not pay for it. Is it any wonder that I consider my BIPAP as one more piece of "Orwellian" technology?

It's always driven Connie a little crazy at how I can fall asleep in just minutes, if not seconds, after my head hits the pillow. Connie's an insomniac, and I worry about that. Medical science has proven how important sleep is to overall health, so I fear that my wife isn't getting enough sleep. I wish I could somehow transfer some of my ability to sleep to Connie. I also wonder if I'm sleeping enough. If I slept any more hours, then my productivity would be almost nonexistent. With eating taking up to three hours a day, bathing and dressing a good half-hour, and getting outside for an hour or two, that bites into the time I can devote to writing or other tasks that I can still do.

I'm not complaining. I'm just trying to express that ALS robs me and others of so much more than body movement. I'm still grateful for the things I can do, and I'm glad to be still alive. Many people with ALS don't make it five years as I now have, and I feel lucky that I'm entering into the territory that only about ¼ of people with ALS get to venture into.

If I don't get eleven or more hours of sleep, my left eyelid droops even more. I've been having trouble seeing out of that eye, and it's much worse if I'm tired –– another reason to sleep. Like so many other things with ALS, there have to be some tradeoffs.

It's good I've always enjoyed sleep and that I mostly have pleasant dreams. I have some nutty dreams like everyone, and lately I've been dreaming that I can walk and talk –– half my life is now a fantasy and the other half is the reality of living with ALS. This is one time that I wish my dreams would come true. But, I'll live with ALS robbing me of time, energy and productivity if that is what it takes to stay alive.

The Cure for Depression

29 December 2018

Most boys have sports figures that they idolize, mostly baseball, basketball, and football stars. I idolized men who made their names in the rock and mountain climbing world. Superstars like Sir Edmund Hillary, Tenzing Norgay, David Roberts, Fred Becky, Tom Frost, Yvon Chouinard and others. Hillary and Norgay might have been the most famous for being the first men to climb Mt. Everest, but the men I admired most were those who put up new climbing routes on big granite walls or on remote mountains around the world. Unlike Hillary, those men were neither well known outside the climbing world, nor were they household names.

Take billionaire Yvon Chouinard –– though in his eighties, many if not most Americans only know of Patagonia, the company he founded.

I seldom admire any billionaire for his money alone, but Chouinard is a self-made man and has done a lot of good environmental work with his money. He also encourages his employees to take a few weeks of paid sabbaticals to do environmental volunteer work around the globe. About four years ago, Connie and I hosted two women volunteers from Patagonia who came to work at the Sitka Conservation Society for a few weeks. One of the women was working as a clothing designer, and the other was a buyer. It was interesting to listen to both ladies talk about what they do at Patagonia. I was very intrigued to hear from the buyer that she travels to Vietnam a couple of times a year to inspect some of the factories where Patagonia clothing is made. She told us that not only does Patagonia pay higher wages than many of the clothing factories in Vietnam, but one reason that Patagonia selected Vietnam was to help heal some of the scars left by years and years of war.

When I recently heard Yvon Chouinard say, "The solution to depression is action," I wasn't at all surprised. Chouinard walks the walk that he talks. I still admire him, even though he gave up big wall climbing decades ago.

Over the holidays I saw several ALS Facebook posts where people were depressed or bitter. Holidays can be trying on one's mental health, especially if family members are not around. Suicide rates, too, climb during the holidays. I don't want to seem insensitive, but Chouinard's words, "The solution to depression is action," kept popping into my head. Since I can't physically talk, let alone yell, I couldn't do what I want to do –– yell through my computer at the people who were posting, "Take action." Unless there is a chemical imbalance in your brain, there is little reason not to try to do something about depression. And, I'm not talking self-medication. The best cure for something negative is to do something positive. A friend who has suffered much of her life with depression fights it by staying active and doing a lot of volunteer work. She is taking action to combat her depression, and I applaud her for that.

When I first started to lose my ability to talk and a good year thereafter, I'd find not being able to verbally communicate made me angry. That anger would spill over to my wife, and then the negativity of that anger would lead to depression, both for Connie and me. If there is anything more contagious than negativity, I don't know what it is. Even though I had not heard Yvon Chouinard's wise words then, I recalled that Will Rogers, the early 20th-century humorist, once said, "If you find yourself in a hole, stop digging." If I kept getting frustrated each time I couldn't talk, my hole was going to get deeper and deeper. I then saw how much more productive it was to see the humor in my inability to communicate. I rarely get frustrated when I can't talk now, but each time I start down the path to depression I do my best to take action and look for humor.

Patienting

3 January 2019

I know I'm inventing a word –– turning a noun into a verb. Please let me explain.

About a half block up the street from our home, lives a man that I'm going to call "Mr. Rude." Over the last dozen years that we have lived here, he often sets off fireworks at all hours of the night. I'm not talking little pop-bottle type fireworks, but the large mortar type that would be reserved for the 4th of July type events –– the kinds that rattle windows when they go off. One of Mr. Rude's friends says that Mr. Rude likes his beer and that he is drunk most nights by 8:00 pm. And, when he is drunk, he likes to set off fireworks. It's not uncommon for Mr. Rude to start around 10:00 pm with his first round, then do another round at midnight. Then when we have just gotten back to sleep, he will set off another round of fireworks. We have reported him to the police more times than you can count and have even had a couple of face-to-face meetings with the Chief of Police. After the police talk to Mr. Rude, things get better for a few months. Then Mr. Rude gets bold and goes back to his normal routine. When his next-door neighbor complained about the fireworks waking up his baby granddaughter, Mr. Rude said, "Well, she will just have to get used to it."

As parents, we set an example for our kids. So, a couple of months ago, I wasn't surprised to read in the paper that Mr. Rude's young adult son was arrested for driving under the influence (DUI). I was even less surprised to see that same son was arrested a few days ago for not only another DUI but also driving without a license. I saw that same kid when he was about eleven years old shoot out a large, expensive picture window with a BB gun. The owners of the window might not have been able to collect for a window replacement had I not witnessed the shooting. Parenting matters.

Just like Mr. Rude set a bad example for his child, some patients set bad examples or are just rude. During a series of appointments at Virginia Mason Hospital in Seattle, we kept running into a woman in a wheelchair that was being pushed by her husband. We saw them in the hallways, a waiting room, and even the cafeteria. In every location, she was being about as rude and obnoxious as I've ever seen anyone be in public. When I ran into her husband in the men's room, I could see the stress on his face. Another time at Virginia Mason, a man was loudly rude to two of his adult children who were pushing his wheelchair, and their stress was evident. He was showing both lousy parenting skills and bad patienting skills.

Isn't our job as parents to set a good example for our children and grandchildren? The answer partly lies in the old saying, "Treat others as you wish to be treated." Why should it be any different for patients? Shouldn't we as patients do our best to show appreciation and respect to our caregivers?

We have all waited in a doctor's office waiting room, 15 minutes, 30 minutes, or even an hour past our appointment time -- enough to test anyone's patience and turn the best of us into grumps. What good does it do anyone, including yourself, to be rude to the nurses or doctors when they are running late? It just adds more stress to their already busy day. A few months ago,

Marcel LaPerriere

I had over five hours of back-to-back appointments during an ALS Clinic at Virginia Mason. By the time I saw the last doctor I was tired, hungry, had to pee and my legs were severely swollen –– my right lower leg and foot were nearly twice the size of normal. Every time the doctor touched my leg or foot to examine them, I would suffer the worst pain I have ever experienced. It was not easy to thank the doctor at the end of that exam, but I did. She was trying her best to understand how she could help and wasn't getting any pleasure out of watching me endure the pain.

Some of the most selfless people I have ever met are people who work in healthcare –– especially hospital nurses. I recall my times in a hospital bed and the compassionate care that I have received and consider it good patienting to do all I can to treat the people who tirelessly work to care for me as best as I can. "Treat others as you wish to be treated." If you do that, then you are a good patient and are exhibiting good patienting skills.

Postscript: After posting this online I had a comment from a father of a nurse who thanked me. Then two nurses also wrote comments. The one comment that genuinely made my day was from a nurse friend of my son and daughter-in-law.

Her name is Therese Hjorten, and she said the following; "I can't tell you how much it means to hear your thoughts on this. One of my greatest sources of burn out is how unkind people can be. Then we have to shake it off, person after person, and go into the next room with a smile on our faces. I choose to look for the good, but it can be wearing. Thank you again, Marcel, for sharing your wisdom!"

After Therese said I could quote her, she said that she had shared my Facebook post with a doctor who also found it refreshing. Thank you, Therese, for making my day twice.

The medical community is like every community –– some good and some bad. People who dedicate their lives to practicing medicine are overwhelmingly not only good people but great people. I could never adequately thank all the people who have helped Connie and me through some trying times.

Why Do I Have to Learn That?

4 January 2019

At one time or another, every school-age kid asks, "Why do I have to learn that?" followed by, "I'll never use that." Then some adult, usually a teacher, will reply with something like, "Trust me, you will use it." I often mistrusted teachers, so I'd stick to "Why?," and then not bother to take the time, or put in the effort to learn what I should have.

In 1969 I was a sophomore in high school, and the one required class I was sure I'd never use was typing. More than once, I asked Mrs. Rickel, the teacher, "Why?" After all, typing is what girls do, not boys. I probably got a D in that class. I hated that class so much I'm sure I did just enough to pass, without doing anything more than just showing up. I was destined to work in one of the trades and I'd never need to type, or so I thought. With no crystal ball, I never could have seen the advent of personal computers or that typing –– nowadays more frequently called keyboarding –– is as important as any of the three "Rs."

Funny, when I was a junior in high school, I figured out I'd benefit from learning to type and that it wasn't just a thing that girls do. In a Denver typewriter store –– back then some stores just sold typewriters –– I bought a used portable hybrid electric with a manual return carriage. The manual return was the strange thing about the typewriter and is likely why it was the least expensive typewriter in the store. Even though it was a bit weird, it served me well through the rest of high school. At the end of my senior year, since I was not heading off to college, I sold the typewriter to a friend who was awarded a fully-paid scholarship to college, and she used it for at least a couple of years.

Though I was such a poor student, Mrs. Rickel must have taught me well, because I never forgot how to properly hold my fingers or the position of the keys. And of all the classes I took over the years, typing has served me best. Even though I went into the trades working with my hands, I don't know how I would have done my work or written the hundreds of letters I wrote to government officials and politicians over the years without the skill of typing.

Because over three years ago I lost the ability to talk, I wouldn't be able to communicate without a keyboard, both on my phone and on my computer. Now that I'm losing the ability to use my fingers, I'm not sure how I'll communicate in the future. I'm lucky to live in a day and age when technology will help me overcome that obstacle. Meanwhile, I owe Mrs. Rickel a big thank you, and I would tell her she was right: I did use the skill. Her class made life easier, and likely more rewarding. Little did I know how wrong I was to ask, "Why do I have to learn that?"

Germophobia

8 January 2019

I have a cold that I assume I caught from Connie since she had a bad one last week. We were both trying to be a bit germophobic by washing our hands and using Purell more often than usual. We weren't diligent enough to prevent me from getting the bug.

Since ALS compromises one's ability to breathe, getting a cold is a real concern. I've read more than one account where a cold lead to pneumonia and that lead to death. So, I'm concerned about getting a cold. But I'm not going to live a life of germaphobia in an isolation bubble. Right now, I have to deal with the runny nose, lots of sneezes and doing my best to cough, which is not easy when one has advanced bulbar ALS.

While suffering through this cold, I've been thinking about a germophobic boss I once had. When I worked for Ketchikan Public Utilities (KPU) not only was my boss, Dick, germophobic, but he did his best to live up to his name by being a real dick. He did everything within his power to make work hell for the six men who worked for him. He wasn't all that bad to me -- because he knew I wouldn't take it -- but also because he depended on me, more than the other five guys, to get the work done. He made up for not being too bad on me by doubling down on the other guys, especially Steve, one of my fellow powerhouse mechanics. Every chance he got, he'd belittle Steve, calling him an idiot, dumb, and just about any demeaning name you can think of. Dick seemed to take extra joy in belittling the guys in front of all of us, and doubly so Steve. A few minutes before our work day would start, Dick would walk into the lunch room and spout out something like this, "Steve, go change the injector on number eight cylinder on diesel number two. Try not to screw it up. I know you are an idiot, but even someone as dumb as you should be able to do a simple job like that." Or, "Mike and Nick, see if you can muster up enough combined brains to drive to Beaver Falls and clean the intake gate for number one hydro." He never talked that way to me, but one day when he was especially hard on Steve, I lost it. I jumped up from my chair and called him every non-printable name in the book. I then offered to take him out back and beat the snot out of him –– not an idle threat since I was a good six inches taller, 60 to 80 pounds heavier, ten years younger and in much better shape than he was. At that moment I became a bit of a hero in my coworker's eyes. And, Dick backed off and was not as inconsiderate in the future. That doesn't mean he no longer got his jollies by being a jerk. On days when he felt like he had to be mean, he'd assign us cleaning details, and we'd spend the day or one time a full week, just cleaning and re-cleaning until we could pass his white glove test.

Dick treated his wife the same way. Worse, he would brag to us about how he beat her up. There is nothing lower than a man who beats his wife or kids. Once when I ran into his wife on the street, I saw she had taken a severe beating and called the police. When the police did an inspection, she refused to file a complaint, and the police told me that unless I saw the assault take place, there was nothing they could do, even though they could clearly see that she had been badly beaten.

Since Dick was a germophobe, I figured I'd mess with him as a way of evening the score, if only just a little bit. Because you had to walk through his office to access the second-floor fire escape, he had to leave the door to his office open when he went home at night. That's because the powerhouse was manned 24 hours a day. I was always the first at work, so some days as I walked in, I'd look for dead flies on the floor or window ledges. I'd then pick up the dead flies and drop them in his coffee cup or on the top of his desk. On days when there were no dead flies in his coffee cup, he'd wash his cup for a good minute before he'd add coffee, but on days when I had placed a bug within the cup, it was a good five-minute washing with scouring powder. And, if I dropped a fly on his desk, he'd wash it for a good five minutes, sometimes with bleach. This went on for about two years, and Dick was never the wiser that it was me who placed the flies where they'd drive him a little crazy. I got great pleasure out of watching Dick freak out over the germs that he perceived the flies were carrying. I never told anyone why I'd have such a big smile on my face as Dick would scour his cup. It was my secret revenge for the way Dick treated the men who worked for him and more importantly how he treated his wife. After a couple of years of me strategically placing flies where they would mess with our germophobe boss, Dick quit, and we got a much nicer boss. Also, Dick's wife, after several years of putting up with beatings, got up the nerve to leave him.

It's funny how the cold that I have right now reminded me of my impish days from more than 25 years ago. I never want to be anything like Dick, but it would be good if I were a bit more diligent when it comes to avoiding anything that will make me sick. I don't want to live in a bubble, but even the common cold scares me because it could literally kill me. Breathing is hard enough without a cold, so I'm going to try to be better about spending more time washing my hands and become a better user of Purell. Meanwhile, I hope I get over this cold soon. It's not much fun.

Marcel LaPerriere

Snot and Slobber

9 January 2019

If you are squeamish about things like snot and slobber, please read no further. But to see some humor in my life, please read on.

I've had a bad head cold these last few days, which is not much fun when breathing is hard enough for me anyway. Besides an endless runny nose caused by the head cold, I've been doing a lot of sneezing. The sneezing has kept me awake at night, and a sneeze is something that's a bit interesting when wearing a BIPAP mask. I depend on the BIPAP machine to breathe when I sleep. I already knew that I didn't much like sneezing when I have the mask on, because it's not a lot of fun having a mask full of slobber. That's especially true when the sneeze is extra juicy, and the slobber comes running down the inside of the mask and out the bottom.

Last night, after a few hours of good sleep, I got up to use the restroom, coughing and sneezing all the way to and from the toilet. When I got back to the bed, I sat on the edge, blew my nose one last time before I put my BIPAP mask back on and laid down. A few minutes after my head hit the pillow, with little warning, I sneezed. It was a juicy sneeze, so I reached onto the bed stand, grabbed a paper towel to wipe the slobber from under my mask without taking it off, which would have required me to sit back up. When whammo, sneeze two and sneeze three hit. Yuk, they were even juicier than the first sneeze. And, even worse, sneeze two must have broken a snot dam within my sinuses, as I could feel a flood of snot running out of both nostrils and also down my throat. Within a second, I could hear and feel snot and slobber bubbles around the rim of my mask including on top of my nose. The snot kept on rushing out of my nose, and soon I could hear the gurgling of snot within my mask as the BIPAP synced with the rhythm of my breathing. There was so much snot and slobber within my mask I became afraid to inhale for fear of inhaling some of the not very pleasant liquid into my lungs.

I had to sit up, take off my mask and clean up the mess. It's not easy for me to sit up in bed and it takes time. I have to reach for one of the four pieces of webbing that are hanging down from the trapeze bars over my bed, and then pull myself upright –– all while trying not to inhale. But the BIPAP machine is programmed to force me to inhale within five seconds of an exhale. So, after the said five seconds, the machine started blowing at full strength, which accelerated the snot and slobber bubbles around the rim of my mask. "Pop, pop, gurgle, gurgle," could be heard over the whine of the blasted BIPAP. As I struggled to sit up, the BIPAP, kicked in the turbo drive. I could hear it yelling at me, "Breathe, you fool, breathe." Telepathically, I responded with a question, "What are you trying to do, drown me in my own snot?" The machine was trying to blow the snot back up my nose and down my throat. Somehow, I managed to get in a breath without inhaling any of the slime. However, the BIPAP was not through with me, and as more and more snot ran out of my nose, it once again went into hyperdrive. Fortunately, I managed to swing my legs over the side of the bed as the machine kept trying to give me all that snot and slobber back. Now all I had to do was hold down the off button for the required two seconds to shut off the machine that was trying harder and harder to force the snot that had come out of my head back in. In my haste, I failed to hold the button for the required time, and the machine stayed on. I reached my hands into the slime ball that had formed around my mask, found the release and as I pulled the mask off, a rush of air blew snot everywhere. My entire face, both hands, my mask and much of the top of the BIPAP machine was covered in snot. It was at this point that I was extra glad that earlier I had the foresight to place a big pile of paper towels on the nightstand before I went to bed. I sure had one heck of a mess to clean up.

I had escaped being drowned in my own snot and slobber and was motivated by embarrassment to sit up and get my mask off in record time by seeing in my mind's eye this headline in the Sitka Daily Sentinel: LOCAL MAN DROWNS IN HIS OWN SNOT & SLOBBER. Hey, you have to laugh when life throws you a snot facial. My three grandsons will sure laugh when they hear I shot snot everywhere — blasted kids anyway.

Anniversaries

10 January 2019

Now more than a week into the New Year, I started thinking about upcoming anniversaries. We usually associate the word "anniversary" with something to celebrate. This coming May, I'll happily celebrate 47 years with Connie. But before then, there are some anniversaries that I will not be celebrating and others that I will, because I'm beating the odds.

It's been five years since I first noticed the symptoms of ALS. Only around 25% of ALS patients live beyond five years, so I will definitely celebrate that milestone. It's now also been three years since I lost my ability to talk. I can't celebrate that. But I can celebrate that, unlike the first year of not being able to speak, I seldom get frustrated and angry about the loss of my voice. The other ALS anniversary that I won't celebrate will come up this coming March when it will be a year since I first had to start using a wheelchair.

In my mind's calendar, I track these ALS milestones by using a good anniversary as my reference point. That anniversary will be in mid-April, when we will celebrate having our beagle, Bella, in our lives for five years. We could have never predicted that she'd worm her way into our hearts as deeply as she has.

I can also celebrate that I'm still eating by mouth. Most people with the kind of ALS that I have would be depending on their feeding tubes more than I am. I should be using my PEG feeding tube more to get my daily nutrition. But even though it is a lot of work to eat by mouth, I enjoy the taste of the food. There's not much joy in injecting liquid nutrition directly into one's stomach, so even with the risk of choking, I'll continue to eat by mouth as long as I can.

As 2019 marches on, I'll face other ALS milestones. I'll soon be getting a non-invasive ventilation machine. As I write this, I can just get by without that machine, but the day will soon be here when I can't. Since there is always more red tape than you'd think there would be to get expensive medical equipment, we started early on the process. When I need that machine to survive, I want it here. It is also one of the last milestones that will happen in my battle with ALS, since I have decided to not go to the point of needing an invasive ventilation machine. I just hope I'll still be here for the anniversaries in 2020, possibly including the first anniversary of needing a non-invasive ventilation machine. If I can make it to May 2022, I'll be able to celebrate a golden anniversary with Connie –– a goal worth striving for.

Concert

13 January 2019

We are lucky that our small town offers lots of opportunities to enjoy great live music, theater, dance, and many other forms of live entertainment. Not only are we lucky to have great local artists, but when some of the world's best musicians visit our town, we get to enjoy their talents at a fraction of the price that you'd pay in a big city. We are truly blessed.

Last night we went to see and listen to classical guitarist Brad Richter play several beautiful and some innovative tunes, including several that he had composed. We enjoyed each piece he played, but our favorite was what he rightfully calls the most famous classical guitar piece ever written -- "Recuerdos de la Alhambra," by Spanish composer and guitarist Francisco Tárrega. I've always loved that piece of music and remember asking Harold, one of our high school buddies, to play it over and over again on his acoustic guitar.

Also, attending an event in a small town becomes a social gathering of friends, much more so than in any big city. Inevitably, we will run into old friends, business associates, one of our doctors, or even the cashier from the grocery store. Since I'm in a wheelchair, and we arrived early, just like on an airplane, they let us preboard into the theater. I pulled my chair into the main row aisle where a few theater seats have been removed to make room for wheelchairs. We then sat for about 15 minutes before they opened the door for the rest of the audience. When they did open the doors, I saw a business associate and a friend of mine, come in with his wife. They came over, and both warmly greeted us before they sat in the same aisle next to me in my chair. A few minutes later one of their friends came in and walked down the aisle just in front of the one we were in. He then turned and asked my friend, how he was doing. My friend responded, "Good, they say I'm in remission and will just need to have periodic checkups." Their friend then asked my friend's wife how she was, and she said, "Much better than a year ago." My friend has been fighting cancer this last year, and after chemo and a bone marrow transplant, it appears that he has won the battle.

When my friend's wife said, "Much better than a year ago," it dawned on me that it is something that you will never hear from a person with ALS. With very, very rare exceptions, no one with ALS gets better. And, in those rare exceptions, many neurologists think that there was a misdiagnosis in the first place. Recently, though, there is promising news from Australia of a new drug called CuATSM that might show promise in not only slowing down ALS, but possibly reversing some of the symptoms. A study of that drug on 32 patients showed positive results. One of my favorite quotes from Carl Sagan is, "Extraordinary claims require extraordinary evidence," and to me, a study with just 32 patients doesn't seem like extraordinary evidence. Also, was the study a double-blind study? And what other prejudices might have biased the study? I'm hopeful, but there must be scientific proof beyond one study of 32 people. Hopefully, the study will be replicated with positive results, and more extraordinary evidence will come forth.

As a person living with ALS, it's easy to withdraw within one's self. That is why, despite the risk of picking up another cold or some other sickness, I'll continue to get out of the house and attend public events. The risk of catching something is less than the risk of depression that could come from isolation -- especially in our northern climate where this time of year there is so much darkness. Cabin fever can easily overcome anyone who doesn't make an effort to fight it. And, speaking of darkness, I sure hope the new drug CuATSM will help shed some light on a cure and give hope to the thousands of people who are fighting ALS worldwide.

Marcel LaPerriere

A Bear Nearly Killed Me

20 January 2019

It's winter, and bears are supposed to be hibernating, but bears will get out of their dens and roam around, even in the dead of winter. When I worked for Ketchikan Public Utilities, (KPU) I'd often fly in a helicopter to the Silvis power plant, an unmanned and remote powerplant that sits in an avalanche-prone valley. On days when there was a high overcast or clear skies, we'd fly over the tops of the mountains and over Upper Lake Silvis to reach the hydroelectric power plant. On those days we'd sometimes see black bears out wandering around on the snow, or even on the frozen upper lake. In the dozen winters that I flew to Silvis power plant, I averaged seeing around two or three bears each winter. And that doesn't count the many times we'd see bear tracks when backcountry snowshoeing during the winter. Anyway, just because it's winter doesn't mean you are safe from seeing a bear in the wilds of Alaska.

Over the many years I've explored the mountains of Alaska, we have always joked that the best defense from a bear attack is to be able to outrun the person who you are hiking with. For many years I could easily outrun Connie. That's why she always carried the bear spray, and I didn't. Now that I'm confined in a wheelchair, and even though my power wheelchair can go 5 miles per hour, Connie and Bella can outrun me. So I'm now the one going to get eaten, and not Connie or our little dog, if we encounter a bear in Sitka National Park, or on the cross trail.

The bear attack that nearly did me in yesterday evening had more to do with my ALS, especially since the bear that almost got me was an extra cute fictitious bear. As we sat comfortably in our living room, and a little beagle did everything she could to protect us through endless distractions, we watched Paddington 2, and the laughter nearly did me in. My breathing has become so compromised that laughter literally takes my breath away. Then, because ALS also makes me extra emotional, I cried at the tenderly sweet ending of the movie. It's true. That cute little bear named, Paddington nearly did me in. I should have known better than to watch Paddington 2, because we had watched the first Paddington movie a couple of weeks ago. But even with what is now two warnings, if a Paddington 3 comes out, I'll be the first in line to see it. Dying laughing would be one heck of a way to go.

Staying Positive — Luck vs. Work

25 January 2019

In recent days, in light of the fact that I have ALS, I've been asked a couple of times how I stay positive. I've answered that there is no one magic bullet. Maybe I should have answered, hard work and luck.

I remember once hearing that "Good luck is 10% chance and 90% work." I don't totally agree with that. Sometimes "luck" can be contributed to work, but at what ratio? Take the house we live in. I feel darn lucky that we live where we do. That the land where we built happened to come on the market when it did was just pure luck. However, it took hard work to earn the money to buy the land, and even harder work to build the house. I look back with happiness and pride, knowing that it took a lot hard of work to achieve our goal of building what many would consider a dream house. But I'd chalk it up to pure luck that I'd recently learned a technique to build the foundation that made the house affordable. Several other people who wanted to build on the land didn't know about the method and therefore didn't buy the land in the first place. Both Connie and I had more than full-time jobs when we took on building, knowing what also made the project affordable was our sweat equity and our endless hours of hard work that it took to gain that equity. We were darn lucky that our son, Zach, helped us build the house. So, what was the ratio of luck versus hard work? I don't know.

Much the same, what ratio of work versus luck tempers my positive attitude? I'm darn lucky to have the wife and family that I have and to live where we do. Both our house and the town we live in go a long way to making me happy. The last few days, right out our front windows at lake shore, I have been able to watch several bald eagles bathing. How can I not be uplifted as they dip themselves into the lake, splashing water that often glistens in the sun, and then spreading their wings to dry while sitting on our dock? Or on our daily walks as I cruise along in my power wheelchair on the Seawalk, when I see a little playful sea otter lying on its back in the water with what looks like a big smile on his face. Across the channel I might see a humpback whale spout just seconds before waving its tail in the air as it descends below the waves. I see beautiful snow-capped peaks, knowing not too many years ago I stood on top of many of them. Even our walks in the forest of magnificent hemlock and spruce trees –– how can I not be uplifted by what nature places in front of my eyes?

A lot of one's attitude has to do with how one perceives things. Many years ago we took our friend Roger, and his family out for an afternoon of sailing on the waters near Ketchikan, Alaska. Besides Roger, his wife Penny, and their three kids, we had on board Roger's brother and his wife who were visiting Alaska from Southern California. As we motored Terra Nova out of the harbor on a perfect day for sailing, it was easy to see that though Roger's brother was having the time of his life, his wife wasn't. She was sitting down in the cabin and not up on deck like the rest us who were enjoying the glorious sunny day. Up the channel a little way when it was time to lift the sails, the wife popped her head out of the companionway with an amazingly big smile on her face. She was smiling because she heard the word "sale," not "sail," and assumed we were going shopping. When we said we were not going shopping but putting up sails to enjoy the power of nature, she almost started crying, went back below and pouted. What should have been a beautiful afternoon of three to four hours of sailing was cut to about a half hour because her bitterness spilled over, ruining the day for the rest of us. On that day I bet a million Californians would have given anything to be in Alaska sailing on a beautiful afternoon with beautiful scenery in all directions. Sadly, she could only see the beauty in material things to shop for, and not the beauty that Mother Nature was giving us for free. And minutes before we lifted the sails, we were watching a black bear on the beach. It was a perfect day, but that lady couldn't have cared less. And I surmise if that woman is ever forced to confront a disease like ALS, she will be as bitter about it as she was about sailing that day. "Sometimes we need to stop and smell the roses." On that day, we needed to appreciate what was put right in front of us.

Work, luck, and how one perceives things has a lot to do with how one feels. I hate everything about ALS, but know that I'm blessed to have the family that I do, and that I live where we do. The rest of humanity is not as lucky as I am. I have a roof over my head, I can afford to eat, I'm not living in a war zone with people shooting at me, and I'm not a refugee –– the list could fill many pages.

How do I stay positive? Luck, work, and my perception of life. It's not easy to forget that ALS has robbed me of my ability to talk, walk, and many other things. But what is to be gained by being bitter, depressed or not accepting my fate? Nothing. Until I take my last breath, I'll do what I can to ward off the blues. And the little dog that was bugging me while I wrote this, daily helps me smile inside.

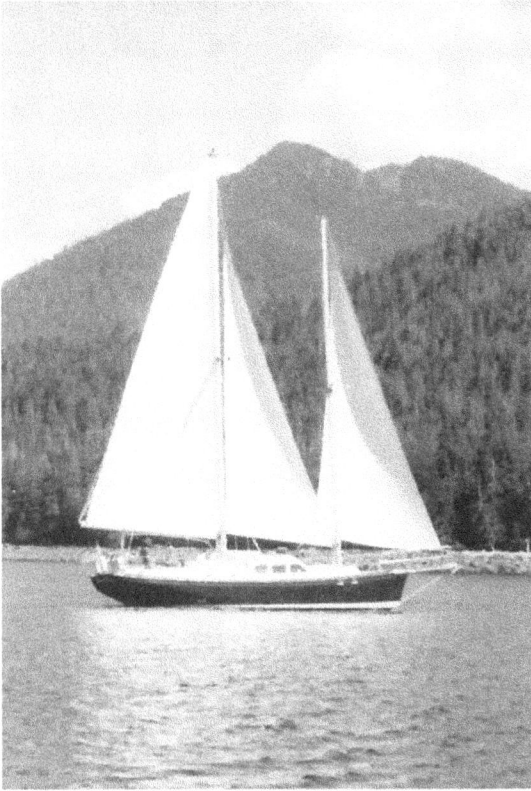

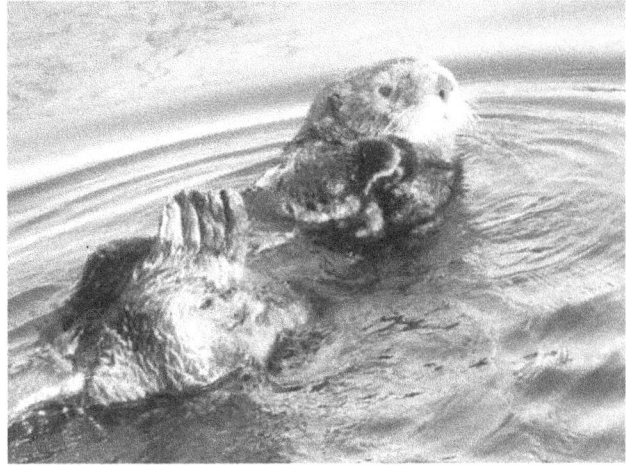

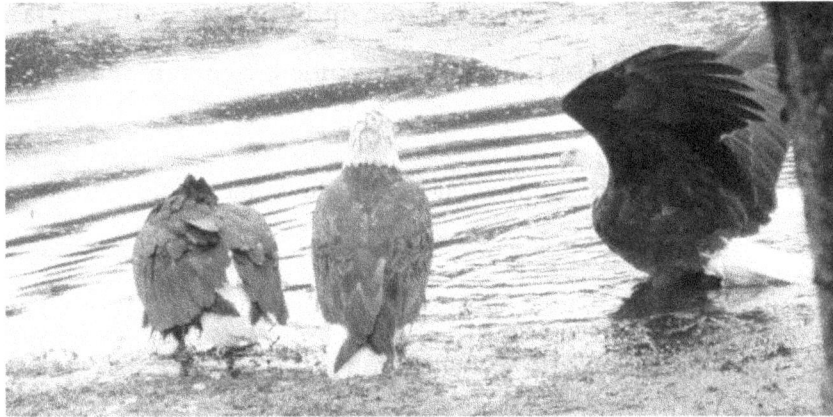

Top to bottom:
1986, Terra Nova.
January 2019, Sea otter in the harbor.
January 2019, Eagles bathing in front of our
house on Swan Lake.
January 2019, Sitka National Historic Park,
known locally as Totem Park.

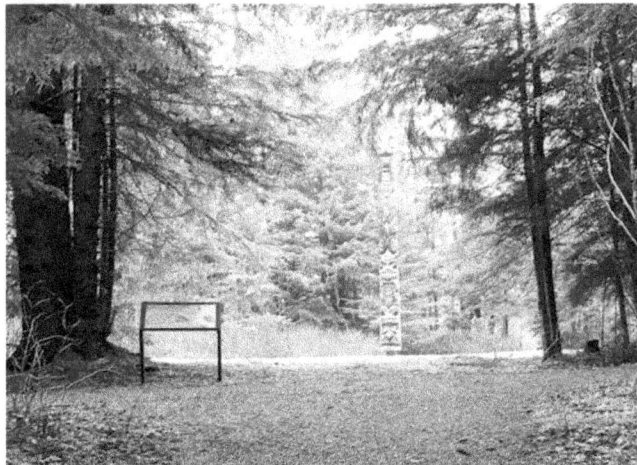

Fatigue, Sleep, and Dreams

6 February 2019

When the doctors first started telling Connie and me that I might have ALS, I started Googling amyotrophic lateral sclerosis to read and learn all I could about the disease. One thing that frequently came up in my research was fatigue, and that as ALS advances, the person will become fatigued more easily. I'm finding that to be the case.

The cure for fatigue is sleep. But even with an average of eleven hours of sleep in a day, I'm always tired. Also, a simple task like dressing myself wears me out. On the occasional day when I sleep thirteen hours or more, I'm still tired. It's becoming a rare occasion when I don't feel like I've underslept. It's a good thing that I've always liked to sleep and that I'm a prolific dreamer.

Even with all the sleep I'm getting, I seem to remember my dreams more than I did pre-ALS. Could that be because the extra rest gives the dreams more time to gel within my memory banks? Maybe I don't have more pressing things to remember?

With a few modifications, one recurring dream features a man that was part of my life in the '70s. That man was Max, my boss at Hallidie Machinery, the company where I served my apprenticeship as a machinist. Not only was he a good man, but it's fair to say that I learned more from him than any other boss in my fifty years of working. The funny thing about the recurring dream is that Max is my boss not only at Hallidie but many of the places that I worked over the years. When I wake up after having one of my "Max Dreams" I can't help but think of him. I sometimes feel a twinge of guilt for never thanking him for being a good teacher and boss. The message is, if there is someone you should thank, do so before it's too late, as it is in my case.

Throughout my entire adult life I've frequently solved problems in my dreams. If I was having a hard time figuring out how to build something, or if I had limited resources to accomplish a goal, the solution would often come to me in a dream. Countless times I'd go to bed with some pressing issue that I needed to find a solution for, and by morning I'd have the answer. Now that my working life is a thing of the past, I don't have many problems searching for an answer. That must be why last night I dreamed a solution to a problem that happened nearly 20 years ago when I was working for a contractor in Ketchikan. The two of us were building a large custom house that was poorly designed, and the owners kept making changes almost daily. When we got to the point that we were ready to put on the factory-built roof trusses, they were all too short to fit the span properly. After a lot of cussing, the contractor realized he'd made a mistake and ordered them wrong. Since this was a large house with a complicated roofline, the mistake was going to cost him a few thousand dollars and at least month's delay to get a whole new set of trusses. This was when things went from bad to worse. That is because the contractor decided he was going to modify the trusses, which is not only against the code, but could have caused the roof to fail. I was not going to have anything to do with something that could potentially hurt someone, so I refused to make the modifications that the contractor wanted me to make. He said that since we were not in the city limits, we did not have to have the home inspected and no one would know the difference. That didn't make what I knew was wrong, right, so I quit. That was nearly 20 years ago, yet last night I dreamt about it, and even more surprising I came up with a solution that would not necessitate the modification of the trusses and would have also been safe.

I have no idea why I was dreaming about something that I'd long ago mostly forgotten about, and my solution is 20 years late so of little use now. Could my brain be working on problems that were long ago tucked away in my subconscious? I have no idea.

Though I've always liked sleep and can't find much good to say about ALS, I have seen one potential benefit. In the past when had a long list of things to do, I'd feel a little guilty if I lay down for a nap. I don't feel guilty anymore, so I'm off to enjoy another nap with hopefully more happy dreams. I might even come up with a solution to some other problem that has been lurking in the depths of my brain.

The 3 D's

7 February 2019

One of the things I love about our small town is the 50-plus nonprofit organizations that strive to make it a great place to live. A couple of years ago, Sitka, with a population of about 8500, had more nonprofits than any other city in Alaska. Per capita, we must also lead the nation. And several of those nonprofits are five to six decades old –– we live in a community that values its residents.

I have sat on several nonprofit boards, and during one two-day board retreat, we learned that to be successful as a nonprofit you need the 3 Ds: "Dedication to Doing and Donating." And the donating part is not just money but can also mean putting in time to raise funds or contributing to the cause in some other way.

What does this have to do with ALS? Fighting a disease like ALS also requires the 3 Ds. We must be "Dedicated" to the cause. We must "Do" all we can to fight the disease. And, we must be willing to "Donate." I'm not using the word "donate" to mean giving money, although organizations like the ALS Association do need cash. When I say "donate," we must be willing to donate time, energy and effort to stay positive. By granting that time, energy and effort we will be happier, likely healthier and probably longer lived. More than once I've watched others give up, become bitter, depressed. One case died shortly after.

By practicing the 3 Ds, others around us, including the ones we love, will be less stressed and more willing to accept our disease. Aren't the 3 Ds an excellent way to show love? If we're not dedicated to doing and donating to what makes love successful, then surely love will fail.

The health of nonprofits requires dedicated people, and to thrive as individuals in the face of adversity, we too must also be dedicated. If we are committed to doing what we can while donating our time, energy and effort, we will live happier lives while facing something as horrible as ALS. Diseases like ALS take so much from us, should we also let it take our happiness and the happiness of the ones we love? No. I'll try to do my best to live by the 3 Ds as long as I'm alive.

Postscript: When I posted this on Facebook my friend, Jo, commented that another "D" could be, "Decision." I agree. She said we are the ones who decide how we face adversity, and it is our decision on our attitude towards that adversity. Again, I agree.

PITA Puppy

16 February 2019

Within a few days of us getting our beagle puppy that we named Bella, Connie was affectionately calling her a PITA Puppy, or PITA Dog. PITA stands for "pain in the ass." And, as much as we love our little dog, she can be a real PITA.

Recently, she has been getting up in the middle of the night, sometimes just to go outside to do her business, and sometimes because she is having tummy troubles. On the nights that she is having digestive problems, we feed her just a couple of teaspoons of kibble and that seems to settle her stomach down. Ever since she was a puppy, she has had allergy problems, and it took us a long time to figure out that she can't eat any poultry. Once we switched to either homemade dog food or food that didn't have any chicken or turkey in it, she got much better. Now, we are finding that she is sensitive to fat -- the higher the fat content in the food, the more likely she is to have an upset stomach during the night. Both the vet and Internet say that if a dog is having problems with fat digestion, feed them small, frequent, low-fat portions of food.

The last few nights, in addition to going outside and her tummy issues, she also wants attention from me. For a long time, she has liked to snuggle up to my feet when I sit at my desk or eat at the dining table. I'm a softy, and it melts my heart when she does that. Now, though, she wants to snuggle with my feet after her midnight escapades, and she will not come onto my bed. That means I either sit on my bed with my feet dangling onto the floor, or I sit in my wheelchair. After petting her for a minute or two, she lies on my feet and falls asleep. That might be good for her sleep quality, but it's not so very good for mine. How can I refuse a little dog that comes to my bedside, cries, and just wants to have a little affection? I can't, especially when I see how happy it makes her. Yes, she is a PITA.

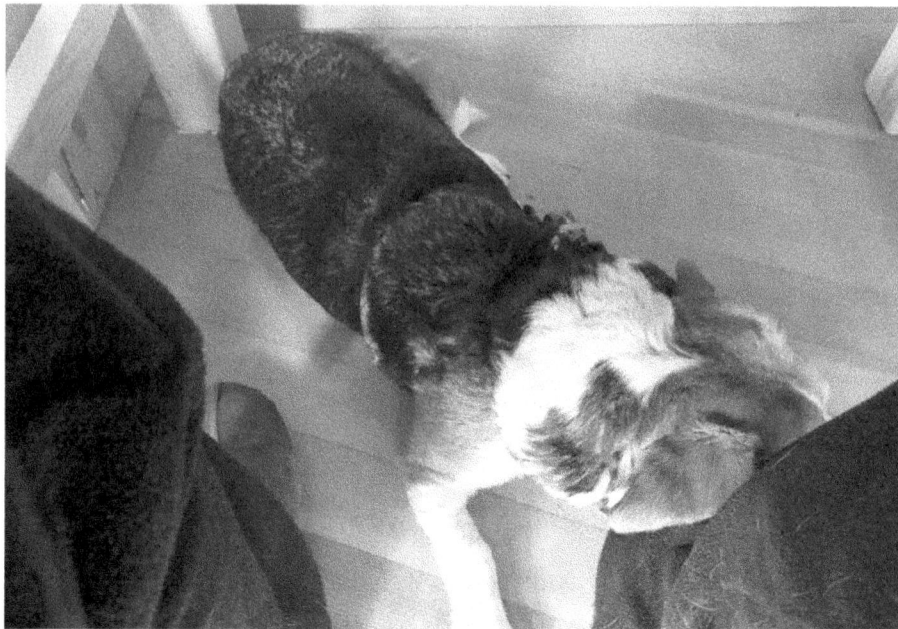

2019. Bella sleeping on my foot while I work at my desk.

As ALS progresses, fatigue also becomes more and more of a factor –– hence the need for more and more sleep. As of this date, I need eleven or twelve hours of sleep in a day. Part of what helps keep my spirits high is a PITA Puppy named Bella. I just wish she'd come up on my bed, and then we'd both be happy. Last night I tried to sleep in my wheelchair, but that didn't work, and neither did a bribe with a treat, to coax her back into Connie's bed, which sits right next to my hospital type bed. By the time I gave up, I was wide awake, so I rolled out to my computer around 1:00 am, and Bella was happy to lie on my feet for all of 30 seconds before heading to the couch to sleep –– a real PITA. Said full of affection for a little loving dog.

Glide Slope

22 February 2019

I always wanted to learn to fly a plane. I suppose the thought of seeing the world from a bird's eye view was something to get excited about. However, I also knew of all the leisure activities that one can partake in, flying might be the most expensive of them all. Since I was already enjoying sports like sailing and scuba diving, it was apparent that flying wasn't something I could afford. Then, during a routine eye exam, the eye doctor told me that I had some of the worst stereo vision that he'd ever seen. Since I'd never heard of stereo vision, I asked him what that meant, and he told me that it was just a fancy way of saying, "depth perception." He went on to say, "I bet you have a hard time parallel parking a car." How right he was. Well, with poor depth perception, I figured that flying was out. After all, if you can't tell how far you're off a runway while landing, then maybe it's not a very good idea to take up flying anyway.

So I know almost nothing about flying, but I do know that the glide slope ratio is about an airplane's ability to glide without power. For instance, the Boeing 737-300, which for many years was the workhorse of the skies here in Alaska, has a glide slope ratio of around 17:1. In other words, for every 17 feet forward the plane will descend one foot when gliding without power. I also know that ALS is about as different from flying as a sewing machine is to a bandsaw. However, since the one given with ALS is that there will almost always be a further decline, it seemed to me that a glide slope analogy chart was a good way to demonstrate my various declines.

Please let me regress for a minute. Several years ago, one pleasant afternoon, I was in Colorado walking on the upper northwest reaches of my brother Fred's ranch south of Denver, about a mile from where the Front Range Mountains rise from the foothills. As I walked, I heard a strange noise that I could not identify, a sort of a whooshing sound that didn't make any sense. Soon I saw a moving shadow on the land. It was a glider soaring less than a hundred feet above the ground, westbound into an ever-rising hill. The pilot and I waved at each other; though he looked to be close enough that I could have shaken his hand. As I was trying to figure out where he was going to land, the glider banked, slightly dipping its left wing in what I'd think was too close for comfort, because it was just a few feet off the scrub oak trees that dot the land between patches of dried yellow grazing grass. I watched in fascination as it glided past, and a little to my surprise, instead of descending, started gaining elevation. I watched the glider gain more and more elevation, and by the time it was nearing the edge of my visual range, the pilot had taken advantage of the thermal currents prevalent along the Front Range, to guide the glider to well over 2000 feet in elevation.

What I thought was going to be a landing of the glider, or even a crash, ended up being saved by the afternoon thermals and an obviously skilled pilot. Gosh, if it was only that easy to find a drug or some other therapy that worked liked a thermal to reverse the decline of ALS. But there isn't, and in my case, any improvements in symptoms are always short lived. It's probably safe to say somewhere around 99% of people living with ALS would say the same.

Glideslope

SCALE: 0 TO 10

12
10
8 — Eyes
6 — Walking
4 — Eating — Hands — Breathing
2
0 — Speech — Drinking

2014   2015   2016   2017   2018   2019   2020

YEARS FROM ONSET: INCLUDING PROJECTION INTO NEXT YEAR

——Speech ——Eating ——Drinking ——Walking ——Breathing ——Hands ——Eyes

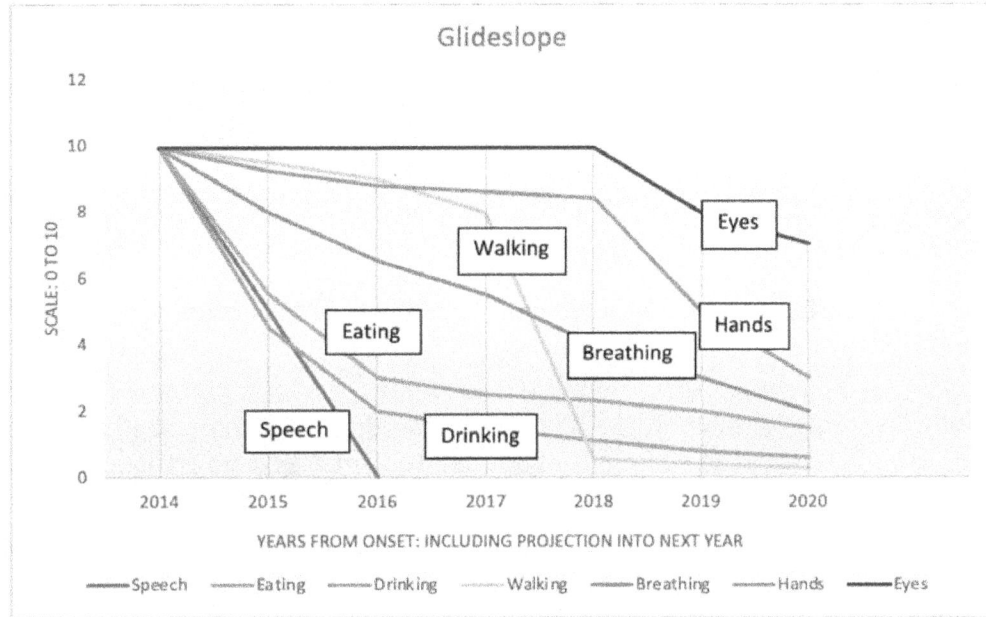

Back to the glide slope analogy chart. All the chart lines start in 2014 because that was the first year I started noticing a decline. Like many people with ALS, it's not always easy to put the finger on the early signs of ALS, and I very well might have had symptoms in 2013. I'm just not sure.

I have labeled the first symptom, "Speech," because I noticed that I was having trouble with speech first. Also, speech was the first thing on the line chart that reached the "0" level of decline. In just two short years I went from a booming voice that some had called a "radio voice" to no voice at all. At first, losing my ability to talk was extra frustrating and depressing, but now I've learned to laugh at it. Just a few days ago I was sitting in my power wheelchair inside our van, waiting for Connie to come out of the hardware store, when I saw one of my former employees walking by. When Connie came back out of the store, she asked, "Did you see Robert?" I then typed into my phone, and then hit, "Talk," so that Connie could hear, "Yes, I was going to yell at him, but he got in the door before I had a chance." We both laughed knowing full well there was no way I could have yelled, or even verbally said "Hi."

The "Eating" and "Drinking" symptoms on the line chart are similar, but different, too. I can't eat like most people do, but I can still eat moist and soft foods via the mouth. However, drinking thin liquids like water is getting almost impossible. I do have a feeding tube, and I could get my hydration and nutrition via the tube, but it's not much fun to have liquid nutrition pumped through a tube directly into my stomach. So, even with the extra risk of choking, I'll continue to get both hydration and nutrition via my mouth. However, to get enough hydration, I need to eat foods that contain a lot of water, like applesauce, hot cereal and of course, my favorite, ice cream.

"Walking" is next on the line chart. I've often said that for me this decline has been much like walking down a set of stairs, some with landings and sometimes, jumping down two stairs at once. But, when I lost my ability to walk, it was like jumping off a two-story balcony, it was so rapid. I had been having balance problems, but I never thought I'd be walking with the assistance of a walker and the next day be confined to a wheelchair. I'm happy to report that I can still walk a few feet with a walker, but when I walk, it's a bit like walking with legs that more closely resemble half-cooked spaghetti noodles, rather than human legs.

"Breathing," the next line on the chart, is the most important. Sadly, it's the failure of the diaphragm muscle resulting in the inability to breathe, which causes most deaths in people living with ALS. So I'm going to do all I can to keep that line on the chart from hitting zero for as long as I can.

The next to the last line is "Hands." Since I have some sort of bulbar onset ALS, I thought I'd be spared the loss of mobility in my hands. How wrong I was. So far, the loss of dexterity is mostly confined to my left hand, and that is good because I'm right-handed. More and more typos and slower typing caused me to notice the decline in hand function. I could do a whole chart just on my left hand because even though I'm losing function in that hand, my typing is better now than it was a couple of months ago. My brain must be learning to adjust to make up for the loss of fine motor function required to type.

The last line is "Eyes." When I could find very little about eyes being affected in information about ALS, I posted this question on two different Facebook ALS Support sites: "Is anyone else having problems with eyesight?" I was a little surprised at how many people responded that they were. It seems that, like me, many ALS sufferers are having trouble keeping their eyelids open. Hence the problem with eyesight. In my case, it's my left eyelid that doesn't want to stay open. I'm finding that if I'm a little tired, that eyelid gravitates shut. And when I wake up in the middle of the night, I often have to use my fingers to pry open that eye. My right eye opens fine, but not my left eye. During the day this causes problems because my left eyelashes partially block my vision. Luckily, I've found the cure is just to get more sleep. If I'm well rested, this seems to be less of an issue. I'm told that an eye lift surgery called blepharoplasty might help. If I have that surgery, I might actually be able to have one line on the chart that heads up, instead of down.

The chart was already crowded enough, or I might have added things like "Attitude" or "Happiness." For sure the "Attitude" line would have shown an upward tendency. And, possibly "Happiness" would have also shown a rising trend.

Since February is my birth month, I'll try to update the chart each year around my birthday, if for no other reason than to visualize the downward trends not always easily seen. As of this date, I hope to add many more years to the chart. I should possibly also chart all the things that are positive in my life. If I did that, the positive chart would totally outshine the Glide Slope chart.

Close Calls

23 February 2019

A few days ago, a Facebook friend who lives in England posted a video that featured some lucky people who had some very close calls and barely missed bodily harm or death. One of the clips showed a very fast racing sailboat coming within inches of hitting a woman who was standing in an inflatable dingy. In the clip the sailboat was making a 180-degree turn. First, the long bowsprit nearly hit the woman, and then the boat did a power slide. Then the stern almost hit her before the boat sped off in the opposite direction from which it had come. A similar thing happened to us many years ago as we were sailing at breakneck speed in our sailboat Terra Nova.

For most people living with ALS, close calls become a way of life. They sure have for me. Because my ALS started within the bulbar region of my brain, not only did I lose my ability to talk, but swallowing has become a real issue. This means I frequently choke on food, water, and even my own saliva. Fortunately, I've learned to minimize the choking after way too many close calls. Not being able to breathe and nearly passing out while choking is not much fun.

The Adventure Continues

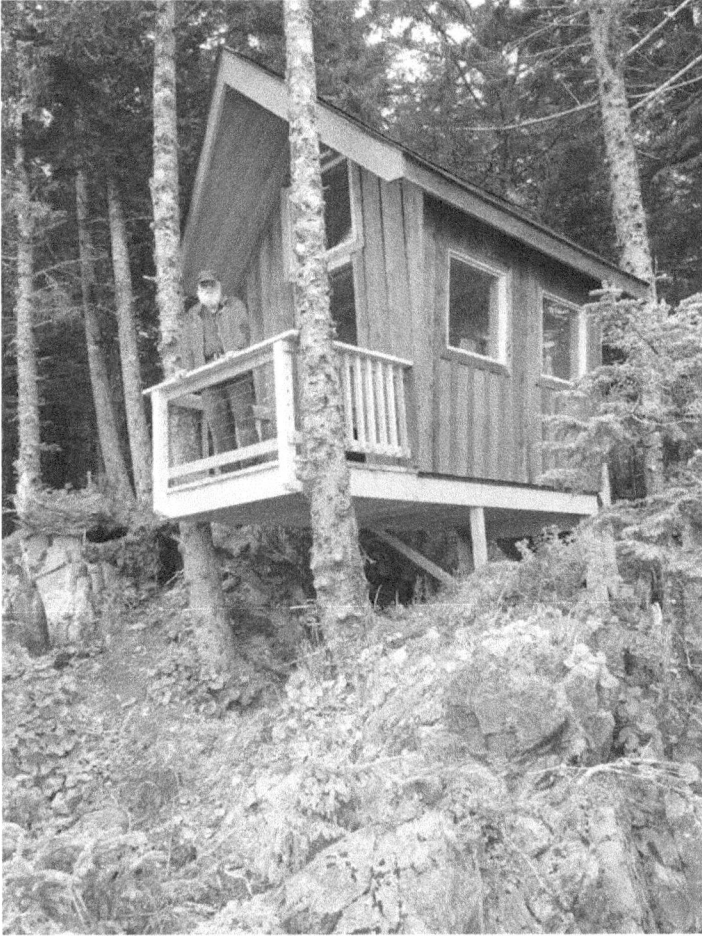

2014. I'm standing on the front deck of the tea-house, treehouse that I designed and built with the help of my wife, Connie, son, Zach, my grandson, Blake and the owner's son, Torin.

And as I was losing balance and my ability to walk, I fell nearly daily, which is not much fun either. In the summer of 2017, I was working with my son Zach and grandson Blake, building a teahouse that was built partially as a treehouse on a very rocky beach. The best word to describe the terrain where the teahouse is built would be craggy –– there was lots of uneven ground with a few rock outcroppings where a fall could be severe. During that project, there were very few days when I didn't fall, and some days I fell several times. I had many close calls, nearly falling off the rocks where I could have gotten myself badly hurt. Fortunately, most of my falls were on the soft ground, but once, though I fell about three feet off a rock and landed on my shoulder, I was able to roll onto my back and was not hurt. Pun intended –– that fall qualified easily into the close-calls category.

Nowadays, I'm mostly confined to my wheelchair, but I do use a walker to walk from my bed to the bathroom, about the length of three beds. When I get up at night to use the toilet, it's unusual not to have at least one close call coming or going from my bed to the bathroom. I just try my best not to fall, and so far, I haven't. It's the same getting in and out of the shower –– lots of close calls, but no falls yet.

In my power wheelchair, I've had several close calls, maybe none more so than a couple of days ago. For a change in scenery I wanted to go to a different location than we usually do, so we decided to see if I could get up the trail to Thimbleberry Lake. The trail had a little ice on it, but enough gravel was poking through the ice that the chair was making it up the hills okay. Then came a section of the trail that is not as steep, but with a small ditch running across it, and worse, a right sloping terrain of about 15 degrees. Neither the ice, the ditch nor the 15° slope would cause danger going up the hill, but what worried me was coming back down. I'd have to be careful on that spot and a few more. After a pleasant trip to the lake we headed back down to the van, and when I got a good look at the worrisome spot from the uphill vantage point, I questioned my sanity for going over it. But I preceded with great care. When I came to the ditch, the left front wheel on my power wheelchair fell into it, and the chair with me in it lurched forward and to the left. If I hadn't been seat belted in, I might have been catapulted out of the chair. For just a second, the chair came up on just that one wheel. I thought the chair and I were going to roll forward and flip onto my left side. Another close call, and for sure, an adrenalin generator.

Before telling the story of the close call in our sailboat, here's the condensed version of the events leading to it.

In 1986 we launched Terra Nova, a custom-designed and built steel schooner. The hull was designed by Grahame Shannon, who in my opinion was one of the best yacht designers of that time, and built by Dieter Pollack, one of the best steel sailboat builders. Both men lived and worked in Vancouver, B. C., so that is where the hull of Terra Nova was built. To afford Terra Nova, we had to finish the interior of the boat ourselves and do much of the other work on the boat all the while living on her. (Boats are almost always called "her.") It must have been about 1988 or 89, and we were still a couple of years away from finishing the interior, when another bigger boat built by Dieter happened to be sailing the inside waters of Alaska on her maiden voyage. The owner of that boat, unlike Connie and me who were passionate about sailing, appeared to be going through a midlife crisis. The boat, to him, was a substitute for the sports car that many men seem to buy when they are hit by that midlife urge. And, unlike us, he had the money to buy the boat outright with tons of fancier stuff than we could ever afford. After a glass of box wine sitting on folding chairs in the interior of our unfinished boat and drinking out of cheap stainless-steel wine glasses, we were invited over to his boat. While sitting in his boat's professionally built cabin on plush overstuffed cushions, we drank a glass of expensive wine out of long stem crystal wine glasses. Over that glass of wine and our conversation, I got the impression that his wife was just going along for the ride. Not only was she frightened of the boat, but it was evident that she hated boat life. We said our goodbyes, and as Connie and I walked back to our boat, we both knew in our hearts that, even unfinished, and without all the fancy stuff they had on their boat, we had the nicer of the two boats.

The next day must have been a three-day weekend, or maybe we took a couple of days off work, because Connie, Zach, Connie's brother, Keith, and I sailed out to Misty Fjords National Monument –– too far to go on a two-day weekend. I don't remember a whole lot about that trip, except we saw the largest brown bear we have ever seen. We later found its tracks in the mud and measured one of the hind paws at over 13 inches, not counting the claws. As we headed back home to Ketchikan, we were delighted to be heading back in winds strong enough to sail. By the time we made it to southern Behm Canal, the wind was blowing out of the southeast at a steady 30 knots, which meant great sailing. Terra Nova loved that kind of wind, and she danced on the wave tops, sailing well above her calculated hull-speed of 8.5 knots. I say danced, but in reality, her stern would dig a deep hole in the water, and her bow would lift up, and she would start planing with winds that strong when the sails were all up. When sailing in those conditions, speeds of 10 to 12 knots were often seen on the knot meter. For thrill seekers, sailing in those kinds of winds and that fast is as addictive as heroin. Connie describes sailing at those speeds with that much wind as riding a runaway freight train heading down a steep hill. Every inch of your body can feel the power, and it is true, power is addictive. The other thing about that kind of power –– it's often a toss-up who is in control, you or the wind? That's part of the thrill.

As we neared Point Alava, we could see our new friend on the other steel sailboat coming the other way under sail but heading into Misty Fjords. After chatting on the radio, we soon decided to take photos of each other's boats under sail. We would each sail close to each other and get as many shots as possible. Connie and I came up with a plan to do a 180-degree turn just as the two boats were passing each other. That way, we'd be able to run alongside and take even more great action shots. Just like us, the other boat was also sailing at what would be best described as "hell bent for leather," which meant the distance between the two boats was quickly narrowing. Connie took the helm and I went forward to stand on the bowsprit, an unobstructed observation spot, to snap the action photos. While snapping photos I was, at the same time, trying to gauge when the best time would be to make our 180 degree turn. When I judged to be the right time, I yelled, "Come about." Connie turned the wheel as sharply as she could while Zach expertly handled the sails doing a downwind jibe. To my horror, I could see I had misjudged and had yelled for the turn one or two seconds too soon. We were now heading straight for the other boat, still going around 12 knots. Running back to the cockpit, I yelled, "Let off on the sheets." The sheets are the ropes that hold the sails in position, and if you let them off the sails will flap in the wind, taking away the power they are delivering to the sailboat. While Connie firmly held the helm, Zach scrambled to let the three different sheets go, and Terra Nova went into a power slide with her stern racing toward the other boat. Everything was happening way too fast, but I had time to look up and see the owner of the other boat also racing to the cockpit of his boat, his poor wife's face was filled with terror. Also running through my mind was, if we hit, the momentum of the boats would cause them to roll towards each other, which could tangle the rigging of both boats. That would mean that his single mast and our two masts would likely break and crash down on top of us. It was a near miracle that we didn't collide. If I had a regular wet kitchen sponge hanging on a string and had lowed it between the two hulls, when I pulled it back up, it would have been squeezed dry. That was way too close for comfort and one of the closest calls that I can remember.

After the near miss, I got on the radio and apologized for my stupidity. Funny, in an ironic way, we never did exchange photos. And I never saw him, or the boat again. If we had hit, the accident would have clearly been my fault. As the close call was unfolding, I was mentally calling our insurance agent telling him that the only two boats within 20 miles of each other had collided, and it was all my fault. Later, I thought about how I'd tell Dieter that Terra Nova, our 17-ton boat, had run into the 20-ton boat he had recently finished building.

Like many close calls, the one in Terra Nova was self-inflicted, as was the one where I came close to tipping over in my power wheelchair. Choking on food that I probably shouldn't have been eating would also fall into the self-inflicted category. Can close calls be part of what makes life more exciting and worth living? As a person who has spent a good portion of my life seeking adventures, close calls tend to be what I remember the most. I've also enjoyed the things in nature when I've been engaged in a thrill-seeking adventure. However, would those adventures be as seared into my brain if I had not had an associated close call? Just before a time I nearly drowned while cave diving, my diving partner, Alan Murray, and I came across a baby seal sleeping on a sun starfish sea-star within the cavern part of the underwater sea cave. The baby seal was extra cute, using the sea-star as a mattress. The mother seal was very anxious to shoo us away, and she kept darting at us but never hit us. Would I have as vivid a memory of that event had I not also nearly drowned? I don't know, but what I do know, it was an adventure like the one that made life worth living. And, even with the close call that we had in Terra Nova, the experience of sailing in heavy winds with big seas also made life intense, and therefore un-forgettable.

Yesterday, while taking part in a video conference with other Alaskans that either have ALS or are caregivers, a palliative-care nurse expanded on something that Connie said when we were asked if we had considered moving out of Alaska to be closer to medical care. Connie answered, "Yes, but we decided against it. Marcel says he'd rather live a few months less and enjoy the quality of life over quantity."

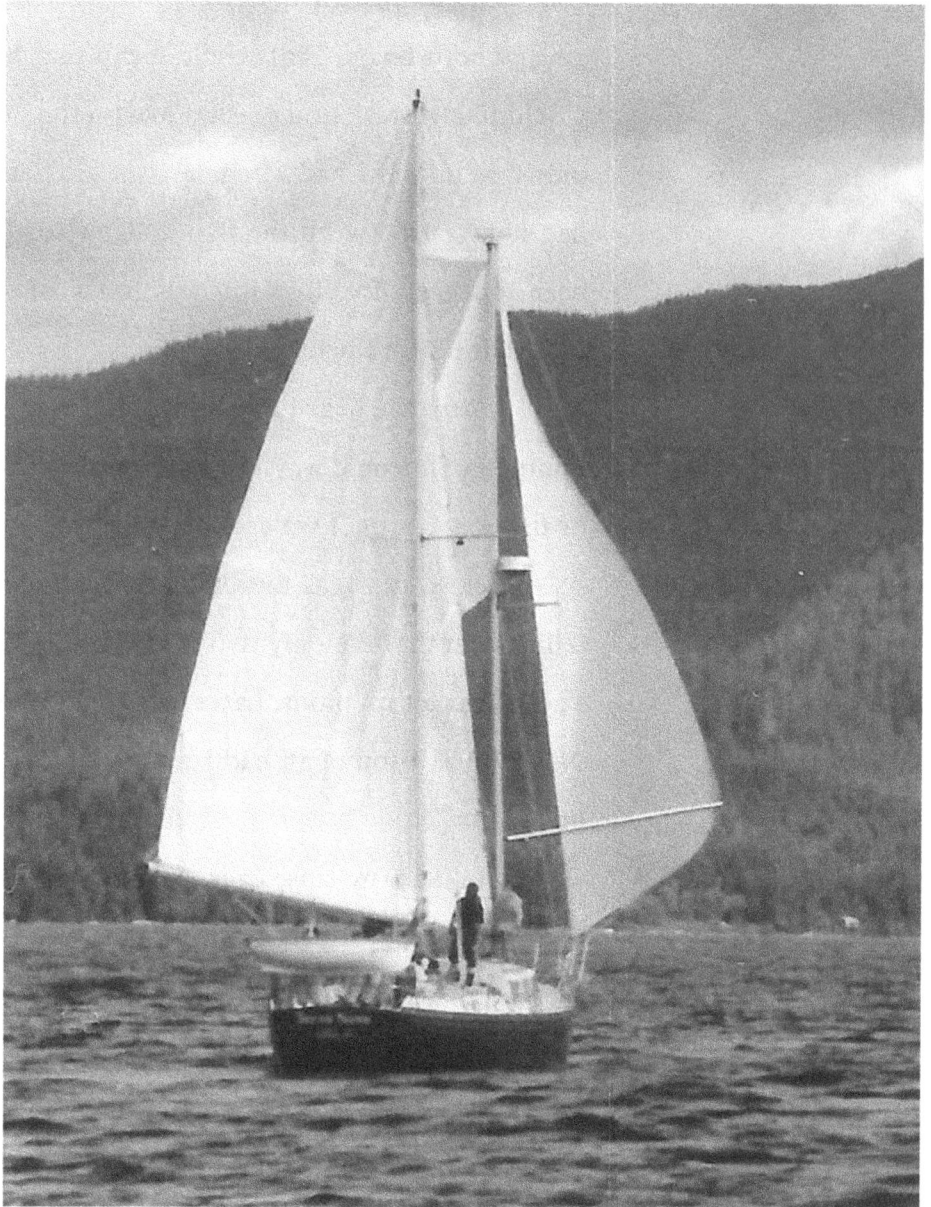

Summer 1987. Terra Nova, sailing, wing on wing.

Then the palliative-care nurse said she wants her patients to decide how they want to spend the time they have left. She said that often their choice is the enjoyment of life over longevity. I'd much rather live my last days happy than to live a longer miserable life. During that conference we were also asked how we don't find ALS to be all-consuming and too much to bear. I answered, "You," because an individual makes that choice. So as long as I can choose, I'll choose to look on the bright side of life. Even if it means a few more self-inflicted close calls.

You can read about the close call in the underwater sea cave in the next few pages.

Marcel LaPerriere

A Tale of Two Caves

23 February 2019 [First written around 1994]

Being stuck in a cave isn't something to be overly concerned about; usually, it's just a matter of time, and you can wiggle your way free. However, if you're 40 feet underwater cave diving, with a finite amount of air strapped to your back, the consequences can be fatal. That's exactly the predicament I found myself in a couple of years ago while diving in a saltwater cave in Alaska. All my diving partner, Alan Murray, could do was watch as I tried to extract myself from a tight spot. Fortunately, my cave diving training came back to me, and I knew the answer to survival was not to panic.

As I struggled to free myself and keep calm, my mind drifted back more than 35 years to my first caving adventures. It was an experience that was just as life-threatening, but I didn't know it at the time.

I envisioned myself as a six-year-old playing with my best friend, Jimmy Hughes. At that age the two of us were inseparable. Our friendship was even closer than the blood brother bond we had initiated by pricking our fingers and commingling our blood. We often shared the same thoughts, which got us into trouble and surely worried our parents to death.

The Adventure Continues

Like most six-year-old boys growing up in the late fifties, we were continually building forts and playing mock war games. We weren't satisfied with your run-of-the-mill forts. No, we needed authenticity, and the endless war movies of that era were our models. We dug trenches as our grandfathers had done in France during the 1st World War and fox holes like our fathers had done during the 2nd World War. It seemed to be natural that we would start digging caves.

Jimmy and I grew up in the middle of Colorado cattle ranching country, so there was plenty of open land for us to do our digging. The place we chose for much of that digging, including the caves, was a 20-foot-deep washout about a half mile from Jimmy's house. The sand in that washout was the ideal consistency for digging deep and fast –– two essential criteria for young boys with little patience. With empty tin cans in hand, we started digging caves about halfway up the embankment of the washout.

As cattle grazed five to ten feet over our heads, we dug parallel caves until they reached a length of fifteen or twenty feet. Then we decided to connect the two caves with a large head quarters room, just like we had seen in the movies. The inner room was big enough for us to stand up and included built-in seats molded from sand. Little natural light filtered in, so our light was provided by candles sitting on shelves that we had dug into the walls. Now we had a real fort, secure from any enemies. Surely it would protect us from any mock Nazi or Japanese invasion.

After our 3rd or 4th full day of digging we decided that just telling Jimmy's parents of our daily progress wasn't enough –– we had to show them. That night we again went home to Jimmy's house and told Mr. and Mrs. Hughes of our days' work. As usual, they complimented us "That's nice, so glad you boys are having fun, keep up the good work." But this time we also got Mr. Hughes to promise he would accompany us in the morning to inspect our handiwork.

Marcel LaPerriere

That night I stayed over at Jimmy's house, and no two boys more anxiously awaited the morning as we did. We lay in bed excitedly talking about how amazed Jimmy's dad was going to be at our superior skills as cave diggers. We knew, as a WWII veteran, Mr. Hughes would be proud of the redoubt we had built.

The next morning, after wolfing down our breakfast, we held Mr. Hughes to his word. The good man that he was, Mr. Hughes enthusiastically hiked along with us. Soon we were talking about the great battles we would fight from the mouths of our caves, and how we would ward off any invaders. Mr. Hughes played along, encouraging us boys to use our imaginations.

Finally, the caves were in sight. We both anxiously looked up the full length of Mr. Hughes's six-foot-six height to receive his approval. To our surprise, he started to tremble and exclaimed: "My god, you boys really did dig some caves." Mr. Hughes just about passed out there on the spot. He and Mrs. Hughes had assumed that the caves we had been telling them about were like the caves we dug in Jimmy's front yard sand pile. Those caves were never more than our arms could fit into, and a collapse would have only buried a few plastic army men.

After a quick inspection of the caves from the outside only, we went back to the Hughes's house, where we retrieved three shovels, and then we headed back to the caves. The three of us spent a good part of the day filling the caves back in, burying everything that we had left inside. Mr. Hughes concerns that the sand caves would collapse kept us from even retrieving the candles and few goodies we had left within the bowels of our bunker.

Both Jimmy and I promised his parents we would never dig caves like that again. But that didn't stop us from doing many other things that were just as stupid and dangerous. Like rock climbing without protection or digging open collapsed mine tunnels. I wonder, do young boys have guardian angels, or for that matter, do adult cave divers?

Now back to my saltwater Alaskan adventure. As I struggled to free myself in the cave, I snagged my weight belt, and it fell off. Then I knocked my mask up onto my forehead and pulled the regulator most of the way out of my mouth. Each breath was about half saltwater and I couldn't see, but at least I was making progress. After what seemed like hours but could have only been a few minutes, I was free. With Alan's help, I got my diving gear all back in the proper places, and we ascended to the surface.

The gentle waves rocked us as we floated 40 feet above the cave. The nightmare of being permanently stuck was now only a bad memory. True to form, Alan made some ribbing wisecrack, and I'm sure I rebutted with one. While we were analyzing my stupidity of entering a too-tight opening, we both concluded that it was a good thing I didn't panic. Had I, it would have been certain death.

While swimming back to the boat, I thought about telling Alan my method of staying calm was to let my life flash before my eyes back to my earliest caving days, but I didn't. It was just too complicated to explain. I rolled over on my back and watched the clouds drift by. Again, I let my imagination drift back, and I saw Alan as a grubby little boy digging caves with Jimmy and me. Somehow, I knew, if Alan had grown up with us, he too would have been wielding the digging can. I even envisioned Alan teaching Jimmy and me how to place black powder charges deep within our sand caves. Back to reality, there was no doubt in my mind Alan was just as crazy as Jimmy or I had ever been. What more could a guy want from a friend?

Marcel LaPerriere

The Good and the Bad

14 March 2019 (π Day!)

I'll start with the good. After more than two years of not being able to move my tongue more than a fraction of an inch forward and not at all from side to side, I'm getting a little bit of movement back. I can now move my tongue easily to the left, likely close to as far left as I ever could, and slightly to the right. And I can now move it a good quarter inch past my teeth, something I have not been able to do for a long time. Will it last, and why am I getting some movement back? The only thing I've done differently is about two weeks ago I started taking 2000 mg of L-Serine daily. Could this be why or just a coincidence? I have no idea.

Now the bad news. Last night I started having fasciculations of my eyelid while I was trying to sleep. The spasms would slightly open my eyelid every second and let in just enough light to make it impossible to sleep. The only way I could stop the fasciculations was to put my fingers on my eyes, but as soon as I lifted my fingers, the spasms would start again. The weird thing is many nights I have needed to pry my left eye open with my fingers, yet last night it was opening all on its own with endless fasciculations. I eventually got in my wheelchair around 3:00 am, rolled out to my computer, and wrote an email.

After about an hour at my computer, I was able to go back to bed and no more fasciculations. I've read about others living with ALS having this problem, and I sincerely hope not to experience it again.

My breathing ability is going downhill. Because of Medicare rules, I can't get the noninvasive ventilator called a Trilogy machine until mid-April, which I hope will be just in time.

Even though the bad outweighs the good, I'll take it. It sounds crazy, but I'm excited about the movement in my tongue. If it will just continue, I'll be extra happy.

Marcel LaPerriere

Bitterness

16 March 2019

"My father ruined my life" is a quote from a man's Facebook post this morning. His post was about his father's ALS and his role as his father's caregiver. It saddened me to read those words and the other bitterness in his post. I don't know the full story, but posting that kind of bitterness will not help this man move on, now that his father has passed. His father certainly didn't ask to get ALS, and as bad as things might have been for the son, they could have been worse. After reading his post, I clicked on his profile and could see that he is in his thirties, married, and has a son. It also looks like he lives in a nice house and has lots of toys, including a jet ski and a motorcycle. From my vantage point, it doesn't look like his life is ruined. He is not living in a war zone or a refugee camp, and it looks like he and his family have plenty to eat. Life might have been hard for him while he was caring for his father, and his father's death might have been hard on him. But the words "My father ruined my life" don't seem to fit.

There is an old saying, "Life is what we make it." Perhaps there are few tests that we will face in life harder than dealing with a horrible disease like ALS, but we still have a choice in how we deal with that hardship. I've probably overused the analogy of war, but I only need to think about it for a minute. As much as I hate ALS, I'd rather be living where I am with ALS than to be living in the middle of a war. Sometimes Americans don't see how lucky we truly are, to live where we do and when we do. There are lots of things that could and should be better, but we should still count our blessings, not hold pity parties and say our lives have been ruined when we are faced with adversity.

As part of the bitter post, the man said, "Do not respond," so I didn't. I would have said that as bad as it might have been for him, the future is now in his hands. I hope he figures out that he has it within his powers to grow from the adversity he faced taking care of his father.

Yesterday I read about an Australian study that looked at longevity in people living with ALS. It found apathetic ALS patients had shorter life spans, and apathetic caregivers also shortened their patients' lives. The results would probably be the same if any disease were so studied.

Apathy and bitterness are as deadly as any disease. A little over five years ago, my wife, Connie, and I watched how apathy hastened her mother's death when she gave up the will to live. Who wants to live a life full of bitterness, depression or any other negative emotion? I don't. Much of how I face ALS is up to me. And having the wonderful wife that I do helps me more than I could ever measure.

DJ

28March 2019

Today was a beautiful day, in fact, a little too nice for this time of year. Because it was so lovely, we decided to take a bit longer walk than usual and to a place I had not been to yet in my power wheelchair. I wanted to look at a yellow cedar bench that my son, Zach, had built from a log that he chainsaw milled and installed along the Sitka Cross Trail. The bench was built a bit over a year ago as a memorial to honor long-time US Forest Service employee John Sherrod. I was interested in seeing how well the bench was holding up to the weather. When Zach and a team of volunteers installed the heavy bench, I was still barely able to physically walk, so I did the little-over-a-mile walk to see the bench in place. Walking back after seeing the bench nearly did me in, and by the time I reached the truck, I felt as if I had just finished a marathon. So rolling along the well-groomed trail today was a little bittersweet, knowing that I was retracing one of the last walks that I did on the Cross Trail. Pre-ALS, this walk would have been easy, but when ALS was robbing my capabilities, it was at my upper endurance level.

Since it was such a lovely day, we weren't in any hurry and stopped several times to let Bella roll in the sphagnum moss, wade in a stream, and jump up on a bench to beg a few treats from us. When we eventually made it to Zach's bench, we were happy to see it looked as good as the day he installed it. Bella jumped on that bench, too, for treats before we turned back. We had not gone far when I saw a man and his dog coming out of the forest. He was carrying a broken off chunk of wood from a recently fallen dead tree, and I immediately recognized him as DJ, a man who used to work for me. He asked if we remembered him, and Connie said "Yes," as I gave him a thumbs up. He then asked if we knew what caused the small holes in the wood that he had in his hands. As Connie told him I could no longer talk, I typed into my phone that the ambrosia beetle burrows under the bark of dead trees and that the small telltale holes are a common indication of their presence.

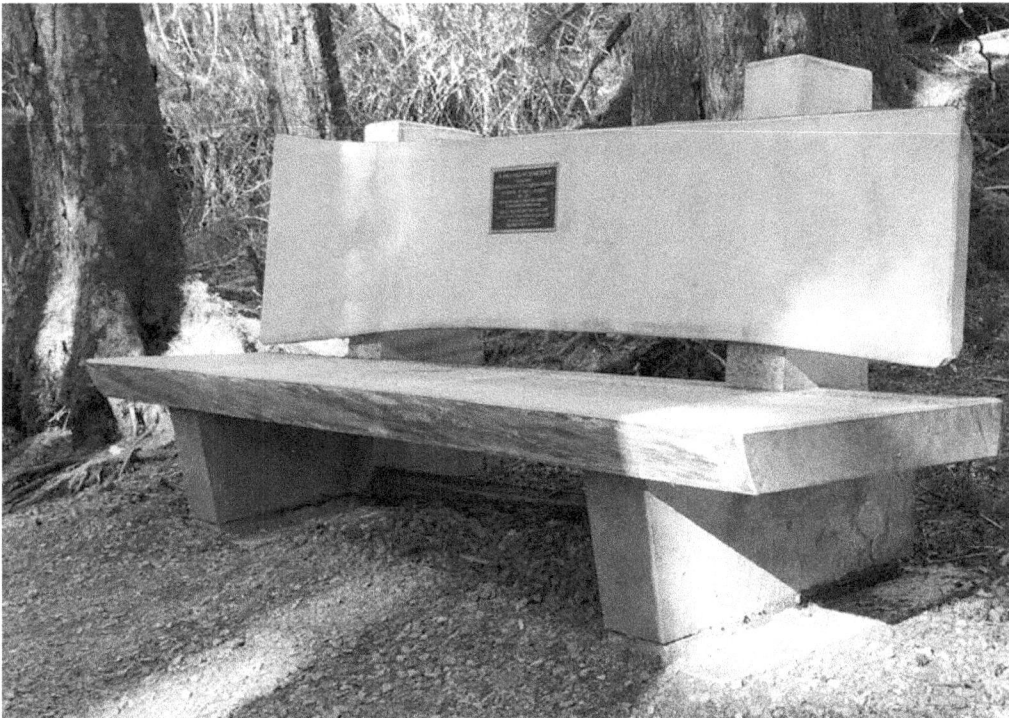

2019. The yellow cedar bench that Zach built to honor the service of John Sherrod.

Nine or ten years ago, I had hired DJ when he was 17. I had done some work for his high school counselor, who called me saying that she had a student who was dropping out of school and was looking for a job. She told me that I'd like him and that she and I, using a little persuasion, could talk him into getting his GED (General Educational Development). I said I'd see what I could do. And I'm extra happy that I did that.

Marcel LaPerriere

From the first time I met DJ, I liked him. He is one of those kinds of guys who exudes cheerfulness, and it rubs off on everyone he is around. Less than ten minutes into the interview I offered him a job on the condition that he work towards and get his GED. I told him I'd be checking with his school counselor, and I expected him to live up to the bargain. I was happy when he passed the GED test about six months after he started working for me. I'm also pleased to announce that he was a good hard worker and learned things fast. Of course, like every young person I ever hired, he messed up a few times and was sometimes late to work. But, unlike some, he always understood why I was upset when he was late, always promised to do better, and did.

Anyway, I was delighted today to see DJ, as I hadn't seen him in five or six years. It was great to hear he is happy working as a laborer at a gold mine not far from Anchorage and would be heading back soon after the winter shutdown. I was even more delighted to hear him say that he often tells his workmates about how much he liked working for me. He said, "I tell them we worked hard, but we always had fun and always strived to do the best work we could." He went on to say many nice things about working for me, and then he thanked me for giving him his first real job. After we talked for a few minutes, he bid his goodbyes and said he was going to take the wood home to show his younger sister and mother. Even when he worked for me, he always liked to share things with his younger sister, ten years his junior. At our work day's end he'd often say he had to rush home to babysit her. He seemed to look forward to his time with her, something uncommon for most teenagers.

Once home, as I drifted off to a nap, I thought about how happy I was to have helped DJ transition to adult life. I was delighted that I had listened to his high school counselor and had not dismissed the idea of hiring a high school dropout offhand. Then I remembered another life-changing experience in DJ's young life –– this one negative. DJ had worked for me close to a year when he told me of an opportunity to go fishing in the Bering Sea. The chance to make some BIG bucks was too good to turn down. I wished him well and finished by saying that there was no way in hell that I'd fish in the Bering Sea, especially in winter. For those of you that have watched the popular TV program *Deadliest Catch*, you will understand why I told DJ that. The rewards of fishing can be high, but it is uncomfortable working on a small boat in big seas, exceedingly dangerous, and to me, not worth the risk. A couple of weeks later, the rest of the crew and I bid DJ farewell and good luck. About a month after that DJ called me from Dutch Harbor and asked for his job back. I, of course, said yes, and with that, he said he had had a bad experience he'd tell me about when he got home and back to work in Sitka.

DJ was part of a crew doing what is called longline fishing, so-called because a long rope with fishing hooks every few feet is dropped to the ocean floor. This rope, or line as it is called, can be over a mile long, with hundreds of baited fishing hooks. There are anchors at each end of a line as well as lines to the surface with buoys attached to it. Once the lines are dropped, they are left to "soak," and after an allotted time they are hauled back aboard where the fish are retrieved. A typical long line boat will have several lines in the water at the same time, and after the soak, the boat and crew will make a circuit to haul, retrieve fish, rebait and then drop the lines for more fishing. This is repeated until the boat is full of fish, their quota has been met, or the season ends. The boat DJ was on was fishing in typically heavy winds with monster seas. While DJ watched, a young man about his age got washed overboard. A few tears ran down DJ's face as he told me with obvious pain in his voice, "The last thing I saw was the look of horror on his face." He added, "I thought about how it just as easily could have been me." That experience apparently so greatly affected DJ that, as far as I know, he never went fishing again.

Sadly, in the kinds of seas they were fishing in, when a person is washed overboard, the chance of retrieving them is about one in a hundred thousand. By the time the boat has turned around, if it even can turn around, the person is seldom found. And if found, more times than not, enough time has passed that the cold water has killed them. Additionally, even if the person is found, it's nearly impossible to lift them back onboard. As I recall, DJ said the risk of turning around was too high, and they had no choice but to motor on.

(When a boat is in heavy seas the skipper will do his best to keep either the bow or the stern facing into the waves. To turn the boat sideways, or what's called "beam to," puts the boat in peril of capsizing. This is especially true if there is freezing spray sticking to the boat's superstructure, which makes the boat top-heavy. When a boat is in extremely rough seas, no prudent skipper will risk the lives of others onboard by turning beam to in order to save one who fell overboard. The sea can be cruel.)

I was glad DJ made it back safe and sound and was working for me again, and I obviously wished he hadn't experienced something so horrific. I hope he is no longer haunted by it. After DJ told me the story, he asked me to never talk to him about it again. I understood that request, and I never again mentioned it.

ALS has robbed me of much, but I feel lucky and proud that I helped a few young people learn a trade, and more importantly, learn the work ethic of showing up on time and doing one's best job. It really made my day to run into DJ, and I'm extra happy he, too, looks back with fondness at the time he worked for me.

Postscript: A few days after we ran into DJ, Connie ran into Jud, another young man who used to work for me. Unlike most young people I hired, Jud came packed full of the right work ethic, always showing up on time, always working hard, never complaining, and always willing to work a little harder if needed. I give Jud a lot of credit for being a good influence on many of the other young people I hired. Anyway, in reference to my first book, Jud told Connie, "Only you and Marcel could turn something as negative as ALS into something positive." That also made my day.

Strolling and Rolling

5 April 2019

I call it walking; however, in reality, it is rolling along in my power wheelchair. Or, just strolling and rolling. Connie and our dog, Bella, stroll while I roll along in my power wheelchair. Sometime during each day, unless it's raining like crazy, I join Connie as she walks Bella. Getting out of the house is good for my mental health, and I love it, too. I love seeing all the things that nature offers, I love to watch Bella as she sniffs her way along our walks, and I love running into other people walking their dogs. What totally makes my day is when we run into our friend Karen walking her dog, Della. When Della sees me, she comes running as if I'm her long lost friend. I've never given Della any treat, so I'm a bit baffled why she likes me, other than I always pet her. Our encounters with Karen and Della never last more than a few minutes, but they are always a joy for both Connie and me. And, I most especially like watching little kids doing what kids do when they are just enjoying being alive.

Since we have spent most of our adult lives living in a temperate rainforest, we are used to walking in the rain, but rolling along in a wheelchair when it's raining presented new problems. The chair controls are not waterproof. The chair gets muddy and often gets lots of spruce and hemlock needles stuck to the wheels and undercarriage. We easily solved the wet controls problem by covering them with a plastic bag. We mostly just live with the mud and needle problem and the mess it makes in the van and on the tile floor inside our front door. However, as we start back to where Connie has parked the van, if I find standing water in the parking lot or on sidewalks, driving my chair through that water goes a long way towards cleaning the debris off the wheels and the bottom of the chair. To protect me when it's raining more than just a little, Connie places a poncho over me and much of the chair.

We are lucky that we have several options for our walks. Our good old standby is Sitka National Historic Park, or as it's known locally, Totem Park, because totem poles grace the trails. We end up there most days, partially because Bella enjoys the trails in the park. She always finds lots of places to sniff, and as a beagle, she thinks she is a great hunter, and there are lots of squirrels to flush from their hiding places. With around

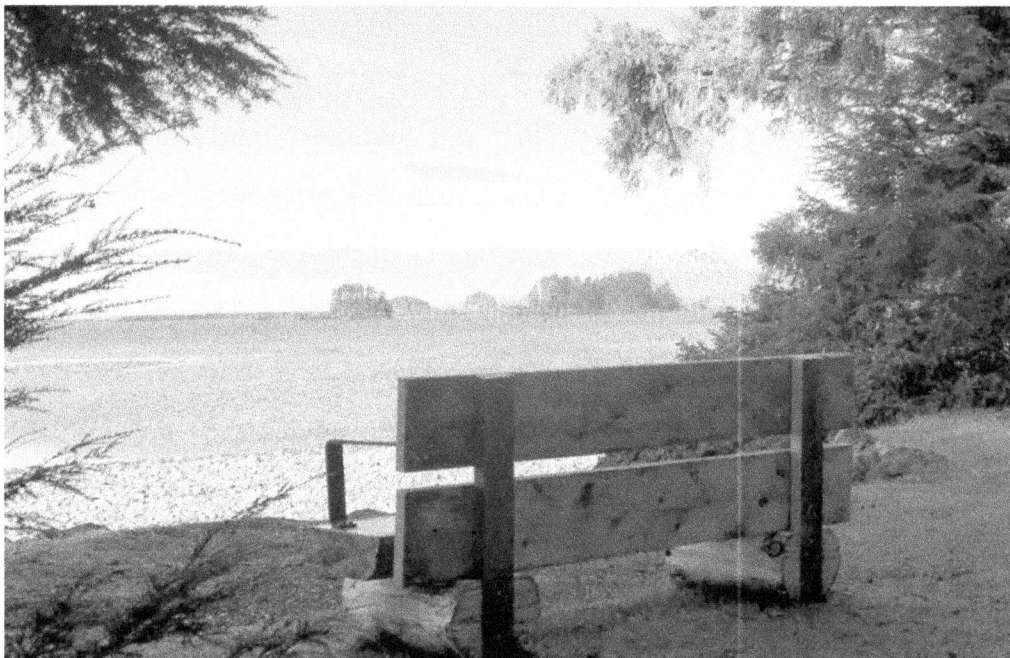

2019. Look at Mt. Edgecumbe and back towards Sitka from Totem Park.

two miles of groomed gravel trails within the park that can accommodate my wheelchair, there is always plenty to see. The ocean side, with about a half mile long beach, is where we frequently walked before ALS robbed me of the use of my legs. On the beach side, there are often a lot of shorebirds to watch, and if we are lucky, we see humpback whales off in the distance. The river side of the park also has plenty to see. Starting mid-summer and going into the fall there are spawning salmon, which bring lots of eagles and seagulls to feast on the fish. In winter, there are often a dozen or more swans in the river or on the shore where the river hits the ocean. And, within the park, there are hundreds of magnificent trees, which are mostly evergreens with a few deciduous trees growing here and there. The deciduous trees change with the season, and as I write this in the springtime, all the berry bushes are blooming. Even though we have walked the same trails in the park well over a thousand times, it amazes me that I still see some unique features on trees. Just the other day, as Connie and Bella stepped off the main trail to venture on an undeveloped trail that my chair will not go on, I spotted a large spruce tree that I had seen before. When I looked up the trunk, I was surprised to see that the tree split into three distinctly different trees just a few feet up, something not commonly seen in Sitka spruce trees.

Since most of the park trails are located under the rainforest canopy, on sunny days we tend to head for the Sitka Seawalk because it is mostly open to the warm radiant heat of the sun. And because we live in an area that can experience what seems like endless rain, we cherish sunny days. We both know the sun is good medicine for our mental states.

Besides the sun exposure on the Seawalk, there is also a new, very nice playground, and with two childcare centers and a preschool nearby, we often see young kids walking to or from the playground or playing in the play-ground. Watching the kids always makes me happy. I take joy in hearing the things they say. One little boy of about four years of age said to me one day about my power wheelchair, "That's cool, I wish I had one." I thought it was cute, even though I hoped that he would never need one, and I for sure hope he never experiences ALS. A different little boy with flaming red hair, also about four years of age, asks each time he sees me, "What's your name?" I always feel bad that I can't answer him. Sadly, each time he has asked, Connie has not been close enough to answer for me. And once, right outside the playground watching kids play, a U.S. Coast Guard Helicopter flew over. A very little boy, that, based on his wobbly gait, had recently learned to walk, put both his arms in the air and as he looked up, he started jumping up and down, yelling, "Dada, Dada." It melted my heart to see such happiness displayed by the little tyke. I assumed that his father is part of a Coast Guard helicopter crew; possibly even the pilot.

Back to the park for a minute. A few Sundays ago, we were heading back to the parking lot when I noted a young couple with a young boy ahead of us. Since they were stopping to look at the several magnificent totem poles within the park, we soon passed them. However, since Bella was in a sniffing mood, we were slow enough that they were soon walking right behind me. That's when I heard the boy that I judge to be about four say, "Whales jump out of the water." To which his father replied, "Why would whales jump out of the water?" In his little, but authoritative, voice the boy answered, "To go number two." If I hadn't been seat belted into my wheelchair, I might have fallen out and rolled laughing on the ground. I chuckled over that for several days.

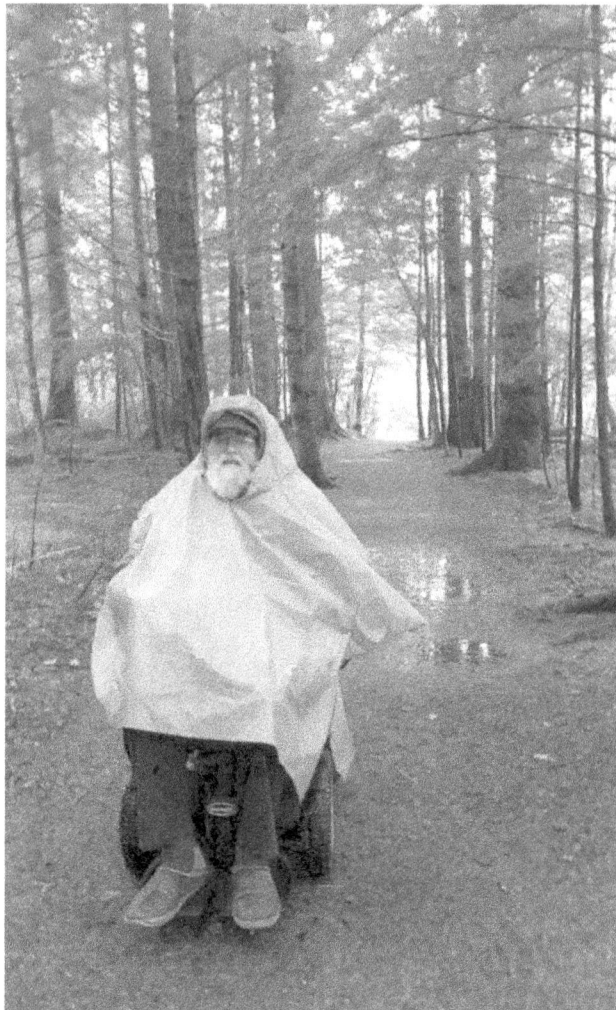

2019. Wearing my poncho on a rainy day in Totem Park.

When we go on our walks, I prefer to roll along behind Connie and Bella. But Bella is mostly driven by her nose, and if there is the right odor, she might spend five minutes sniffing within a small area. So, to motivate her I often zip ahead, and if that doesn't get her walking, Connie asks, "Where's Papa?" Then Bella puts her nose to the ground, and sniffs me out. If I get far ahead and out of view, I like to turn around and watch Bella, zigging and zagging from one side of the trail to the other, with her nose working in overdrive on her mission to find me. Usually, when she catches sight of me, her tail will start wagging like crazy, and that makes me happy.

This morning I was struggling to put on the two jackets that I wear this time of year. I was pushing myself a little harder than I should and soon was winded enough that I vomited on the floor. When I get too winded, my diaphragm muscle is not strong enough to breathe, and after a few minutes, I vomit. For me, vomiting is like a reset button, and that gets things working again. I know better than to push myself like that, but I figured I could tough it out. Wrong! Because of my stupidity, poor Connie had to clean up after me, and I felt bad about giving her a task that is never fun for anyone. As I sat in my power wheelchair trying to get my breath back, I started to think about how difficult daily tasks have become for me. It now kicks my butt to do something as simple as putting on a jacket. Ugh. However, nothing will be gained by dwelling on my losses that seem to grow with each passing week. It's much more productive to focus on the positive, and our walks make that easier for me. I've found that it's important to take joy in the little pleasure in life, and our daily stroll and roll is just that: a little pleasure that pays big dividends.

Marcel LaPerriere

Sitka Summer Music Festival & Stevenson Hall

11 April 2019

Keeping a positive attitude when one is faced with a bad disease like cancer, or in my case ALS, means that I must work hard to keep my mental health strong. Volunteering is one way I do that. For most people, as ALS progresses, the mind stays sharp as the body stops functioning properly. I can no longer do the paid or volunteer work that I used to do, but that doesn't mean that I can't still volunteer my time to do things with my brain. And keeping my mind active definitely helps me still feel valued and part of my community.

For most of my adult life, I have spent part of every week volunteering for a nonprofit or government program that I support. I've always found volunteer work much more fulfilling than paid work. That's possibly because volunteer work is often more appreciated than paid work. Or perhaps it is because you know that your work is making a difference. Many friendships are formed when doing volunteer work, and I feel more a part of my community when I'm volunteering.

As the first symptoms of ALS were starting to manifest, I was just finishing the fun job of building the most challenging house I'd ever built. I was also getting close to retirement, but I'd hoped to build one or two less challenging homes. After that, I had wanted to donate my time as Project Manager on the renovation of an historic building built in 1911. That building, Stevenson Hall, is on the former Sheldon Jackson College (SJC) campus and is now owned by the Sitka Summer Music Festival, a nonprofit that both Connie and I support.

Both Connie and I, being classical music fans, know how lucky we are to have the Sitka Summer Music Festival here in Sitka. In 1972, violinist Paul Rosenthal asked a few of his musician friends to come to Sitka to perform in the newly built community center, Harrigan Centennial Hall. With the backdrop behind the performance stage of views of the ocean dotted with many islands and beautiful mountains in the distance, Mr. Rosenthal recognized that Sitka offered a unique venue for him and his friends to perform works by the great classical masters. The first year was such a success that every year since then, some of the best classical music musicians from around the world come to Sitka to be part of our community and to play beautiful music for the full month of June. When I said the musicians become part of the community, it's because when they are here, they give many free performances during the week in locations like the hospital, the Pioneer's Home, each Wednesday in various cafés, followed by what's called Bach's Lunch, over the noon hour each Thursday. Then, on Friday and Saturday evenings, there are the main events, which are still played in Harrigan Centennial Hall. On Sundays, there are more events, including the free Kids' Concert with ice cream floats after the performance, a cruise on Sitka Sound while chamber music is played, and the ever-popular Sunday crab feed.

For the last few years the Sitka Summer Music Festival has been under the direction of Grammy Award-winning cellist Zuill Bailey. Mr. Bailey has not only kept up the tradition of bringing world-class musicians to Sitka, but during July he and his friend, Melissa Kraut, now teach a cello seminar for some of the top collegiate cellists from around the world.

Both during the Music Festival in June and the seminar in July, the musicians stay in Stevenson Hall. The renovation of Stevenson Hall will not only make the accommodations more comfortable, but it will allow the Festival to host year-round events. There is already talk of piano seminars and the possibility for many more events to be held in Sitka during the winter. As it stands today, the Sitka Summer Music Festival and Zuill Bailey travel throughout Alaska during the winter playing music. After Stevenson Hall is renovated ,there is no reason that the state tours couldn't start or finish in Sitka, which would go a long way to chasing the winter cabin fever blues away.

Besides Connie's and my support for the Music Festival, I wanted to be part of the renovation of Stevenson Hall for several reasons. The former SJC campus is not only an important and historic part of Sitka, but I worked as the Maintenance Director at SJC for the last four years the school was in operation. When the school closed in 2007, many of us were concerned that the historic buildings might be torn down or be sold to a cruise ship company. So when the Sitka Summer Music Festival was able to buy one of the buildings, we were delighted. Plus, of the 40-some buildings at SJC, Stevenson might be my favorite because of my strong association with the people that worked or lived in Stevenson.

During my tenure at SJC, the 1st floor of Stevenson Hall housed the President's Office, and I felt a strong kinship to Dr. Art Cleveland, one of the three presidents during those four years. The other person I liked and had great respect for was the Dean of Students, Dr. David Harrington. Dr. Harrington is an interesting man, in that he worked his way through college as a Volkswagen mechanic, and not only did he earn a PH. D, but he is also a registered nurse, and he is also a nice guy.

The 2nd floor of Stevenson Hall was often called the Widows' Dorm, or Widows' Housing, not that all the ladies who lived on the 2nd floor were widows, but because that is where the majority of the long-term volunteer single women lived. One volunteer, Kristy, had just graduated from college and worked part-time for me and part-time in the student union building as a barista. The name Widows' Dorm had been established long before I started at SJC, and it was affectionately used by staff and students. I say affectionately because, without exception, everyone on campus loved the women who lived there. Though I could never list them all, I can include the legendary Henrietta, who needs to be honored for her years and years of volunteering at SJC. Also there was Duna, likely the most loved tutor of all time. The list could go on and on, naming one dedicated woman volunteer after another.

More about Dr. Cleveland. Of the three presidents who worked at SJC when I was there, without a doubt he was the hardest working, and unquestionably the most passionate about his job. Unlike the president before or after him, he saw the volunteers as assets, whereas, the other two presidents saw them as liabilities. Also, unlike the other two presidents, Dr. Cleveland treated everyone with respect, and he didn't put on airs. Dr. Cleveland and I also had a bit of a friendly rivalry going on as to who would be the first to work in the morning. It was not usual for me to receive an email from him that went something like this, "When I walked to work this morning at 5:00 am I saw your truck parked in front of the Maintenance Shop." Or, I'd fire him an email that went something like this, "When I came in to plow snow this morning at 4:30 am I saw you were already in your office." Since he lived on campus, he would often notice if I got called in after hours to fix a problem, and he'd either thank me in person when we bumped into each other on campus, or he'd shoot me an email. And, he always attended the last formal meeting of each workgroup that was on campus to personally thank them for their service.

Marcel LaPerriere

Being part of the Building Committee for the upgrade of Stevenson helps bring back many good memories. Even better, I know what an asset the Sitka Summer Music Festival is to Sitka, so being part of that team makes me feel valued, and that is important for good mental health. I just wish my physical health would have permitted me to be the Project Manager, but that is not to be. We selected Paul Cotter, a very qualified person, who will do a better job than I ever would have. That too makes me feel good.

When it became apparent that I wouldn't be able to volunteer my time as the project manager, Paul had recently moved from Anchorage to Sitka, so I knew he'd be the logical person to recommend. My only concern with Paul was I knew he travels a lot, teaching classes in various aspects of building science. However, 2019, being an odd year, is the right timing for the construction work to commence. That's because on even years Paul is extra busy traveling to teach continuing education credits that all contractors need to keep their licensing credential current.

I first met Paul in 2008 or 09 when I took a two-day weatherization class that he was teaching over at the University of Alaska, Southeast. Over the next few years, I took three or four more courses from him. Sometimes I needed the continuing education credits to meet the Alaska state requirements for keeping my contractor's license up to date. Sometimes I took them because I always liked learning the latest in weatherization, building ventilation and other topics that might be boring to others but were exciting to me as a builder. I knew Paul had a Ph.D. but was surprised when I found out it was in cardiovascular physiology. I was even more surprised to find out that he also had a master's degree in, of all things, the reproductive physiology of birds. How did a guy go from two totally different scholarly pursuits and morph into one of the best building science gurus in the state of Alaska? When he was teaching at the University of Alaska, Southeast in Juneau, he became friends with the people in Alaska who were exploring the cutting edge of building science in northern climates, latched onto that group, and absorbed all he could. I find it interesting that a person could become so fascinated with building science that he drifted away from his Ph.D. focus to become one of the most respected people in the somewhat obscure field of building science and forensics.

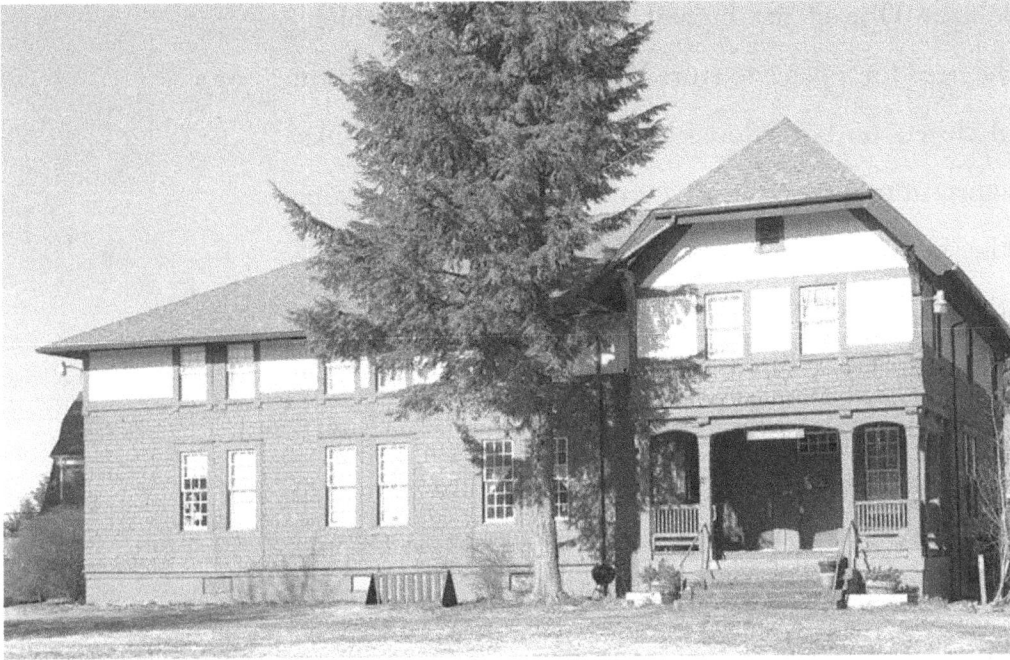

April 2019. Stevenson Hall.

Paul's formal education qualified him to be an observant scientist, and the laws of science apply to buildings, just like they do to any biological systems. Just like we humans depend on many systems to work together correctly for good health, so do our buildings.

I have been honored to be an ad hoc member of the Building Committee, the team that has decided what is needed to turn Stevenson Hall in to a year-round home for the Sitka Summer Music Festival. I say honored because not only are we doing all we can to protect and rejuvenate a historic building, but I've been able to work with some topnotch people. Other members of the team include the Sitka Summer Music Festival's board president, Don Lehmann, a medical doctor who specializes in sports medicine; Dan Jones, a highly respected civil engineer; Jim Steffen, or as everyone calls him, Stef, a highly respected marine surveyor; Don Surgeon, an attorney, and Kayla Boettcher, the Sitka Summer Music Festival's executive director. With the help

201

of Paul, the six of us have done a very fine job reining in costs while still coming up with a design that will function well year-round. The biggest obstacle we have faced over the last four years has been to work with the architect we hired. He has done a great job transforming the interior of the building space into bedrooms with en suite bathrooms for twelve musicians, two offices and a practice performance area. One of my biggest pushes that the architect didn't seem to get was the need for a place to store linens and, more important to me, proper janitorial closets on both floors with appropriate mop sinks. These may appear unimportant to many people, but not to the people cleaning the rooms, especially if there is limited time between turn-arounds.

Besides a properly functioning building for people, one of our primary goals was to provide Stevenson Hall with a modern, efficient, reliable heating system. We had a hard time convincing him to make the building energy efficient. He seemed to be stuck in the past and hasn't kept up with the latest in technology. That he never met a single deadline has been a frustration I would have loved to skip. However, working with the team mentioned above has more than made up for it.

Another controversy, and likely the biggest one we have been dealing with, is over windows. Since we want an efficient building, we decided to replace all the windows with triple pane wood-clad fiberglass frames. The windows we have chosen will be more efficient by a factor of several times, not just because of the glass, but even more importantly, because of how they fit in the walls. The old windows with the old window weights within the walls leak air like sieves. Also there are years and years of accumulated lead-based paint on the frames, inside and out, cost prohibitive to strip off. We also can make an educated guess that some of the glazing compounds contain asbestos, since asbestos was often added to the putty in the years from the '50s to the '70s, another expense that made the decision to go with new windows an easy one to make.

Replacing the windows wasn't taken lightly. We knew that there would be some local and historical agency opposition because Stevenson Hall is listed on the National Historic Register. But, since those that are opposing are not paying the heating bill, it seemed easy to overlook their criticism. I'm not sure that they understand the importance of following the law when it comes to both lead and asbestos abatement. Nor am I sure they grasp the need to have a climate-controlled environment to protect some of the priceless instruments that the musicians bring with them to Sitka. Case in point: Mr. Bailey's cello was built in Venice in 1693 by the master instrument maker, Matteo Goffriller. It never flies in the cargo hold of an airplane; it flies strapped into an airplane seat next to him, and I could not venture to guess what it's worth. And several of the musicians who come each year bring with them Stradivarius violins. One meeting I asked Mr. Bailey the value, on that given day, of the instruments that were in Stevenson. With only a little hesitation, he answered, somewhere between 12 and 13 million dollars. How could we not replace the windows?

Being part of the Building Committee has caused a few stressful moments, but isn't a little stress also a reward in disguise? Because I now live such a stress-free life, a bit of stress reminds me of my working life, and that makes me feel more human. I often seemed to thrive on a good challenge along with the associated stress. Stress makes me feel like I'm not limited by this horrid disease.

A post on the British Motor Neuron Disease Facebook page told of a former primary school teacher who had to quit her beloved job because of her advancing ALS. She was asking for advice on how to stay busy. I suggested she could volunteer to correct papers, lay out lesson plans, or maybe write a children's book. With a little creativity, all of us can find ways to volunteer our time, and despite our disabilities, we can still be productive in our communities. My volunteering has gone a long way to help me not only stay positive but feel like I still have some worth. Sitting around with nothing to do would drive me nuts. As long as I can see and have some use of my hands, I'll volunteering. Now, I must live long enough to see the fruits of all the work we as a committee have put into Stevenson Hall. I'll be extra happy rolling my wheelchair up the handicap ramp to witness the Grand Opening of the renovated Stevenson Hall, the home of the Sitka Summer Music Festival.

Broken Door

12 April 2019

This morning, after we came back from our daily walk, Connie hit the button on the garage door opener so she could back the van into the garage. I saw the door open a foot and then stop, and heard Connie mumble, "Humm," as she hit the door opener again. I typed into my phone that she should go look to see if something was obstructing the door. I watched her walk inside the garage, and saw the door go down and then went back up to the same spot and stop. Connie then came and unstrapped my wheelchair, and I rolled into the garage via the person door. After looking more carefully, we saw that one of the springs had broken, so the door didn't have the assistance it needed to open.

I installed that garage door a dozen years ago, and since I've worked on more than one overhead door, I knew that this wasn't something that Connie could fix. And because garage door springs have the potential to hurt someone badly, I wasn't going to ask either my son, Zach, or my grandson Blake to install a new spring. I typed into the phone to call the overhead door expert, Ron, whom I have known for several years. He always does professional work, and he's honest, something that is often rare in home repairmen.

Marcel LaPerriere

About an hour later, I waved Ron in through our front door. He said, he'd measured the spring and would order a set of new springs, and added, "If I have it apart to add one spring, I might as well change them both. If one broke, it's likely that the other one is nearing the end of its life."

Ron then asked how I was doing, and I gave him a thumbs up. Connie then asked, "You know Marcel can't talk, don't you?" Ron answered he figured it out when I wasn't saying anything, then he added jokingly, "Marcel was always so chatty, I figured something was wrong." Connie then told him that I have ALS, and he asked, "Lou Gehrig Disease?" Connie nodded yes, to which Ron said to me, "Well you look good." And, he is right; I do look healthy. Ron then went on to say that he sees our grandsons walking or riding their bikes around town, and he can tell they are well-raised boys. He went on to say that we were lucky to have them so close, and they were lucky to have us nearby. Connie and I both agreed, followed by a couple of minutes talking about the three boys.

Then Ron told us this story. His 86-year-old mother had been fighting lung cancer, and fortunately, with surgery and chemo, she went into remission. Then they found out that she had a blocked carotid artery and would need to have surgery to unblock it. Ron flew to his childhood home to be with his mom during her surgery, planning to stay awhile until she got better. Sadly, during the surgery, she suffered a couple of strokes which left her partially paralyzed. During the month Ron spent with his mom she kept getting better and better, regaining movement in her hand and then her ability to walk. When Ron flew home, it was with happiness that his mother was getting better with each day.

With that, Connie said that was good news, as I gave the thumbs up. That's when I saw a tear in Ron's eye, and heard his voice faltering. Ron said that shortly after he got home, he received a call saying his mother had been killed in an automobile accident. A seventeen-year-old girl pulled out in front of the car that his mother was riding in. His mother and others were killed, including the seventeen-year-old girl, who was pregnant. He then said, "You just never know when it's going to be too late to say, I love you." As he went on with his shaken voice, "Tell everyone you love that you love them every time you talk to them. You just never know if this will be the last time or not. Life is fragile."

I was struck by all Ron's mother had been through to then be killed in an automobile accident. Then as Ron walked out our front door, I heard his wise words in my head, "Tell everyone you love that you love them every time you talk to them. You just never know if this will be the last time or not. Life is fragile."

Marcel LaPerriere

Marine Surveyors

15 April 2019

Yesterday Connie and I went to the Sitka Summer Music Festival's spring fundraising brunch where the music festival's artistic director, Zuill Bailey, played the cello and was accompanied by pianist Awadagin Pratt. There was some lovely Bach, followed by a glorious Beethoven Piano Sonata, and then, always my favorite, Brahms Cello Sonata No. 1 in E minor, Op. 38.

Since Connie and I are always early, we pretty much had the pick of what table we wanted to sit and secured a perfect location -- one where we could see the pianist playing. A few minutes after we arrived, Sitka Summer Music Festival board member Jim Steffen and his wife sat with us. Since I can't talk it's always a bit awkward for me, but I've known Stef, as everyone calls him, for many years, and I couldn't think of a better person to sit next to. It helped smooth over the awkwardness.

During intermission, I typed into my phone for Stef to read, "I hear you're trying to retire?" Stef is highly respected and frequently sought after for his marine surveying skills. Given that, I thought retirement might be harder for him than most. The intermission ended before I could get a full answer about Stef's retirement. Typing everything on my phone slows conversation, and now that I'm losing hand coordination and having troubles seeing, my end of the conversation is even slower.

Last night in the middle of the night, when Bella woke Connie and me to let her outside, I'd been dreaming about a man named Ed, another marine surveyor I had many encounters with in the past. Talking with Stef must have been the catalyst of that dream. What a contrast there was between the two marine surveyors! I laughed as I recalled this story about Ed.

When Connie and I lived on our sailboat for many years, we were required to have the boat surveyed every three or maybe four years. It was always a joke and upset me that we had to toss money out the window for this required survey. We knew our boat better than any marine surveyor could, since we had built it from the hull up. Even more disturbing was that any junior high school kid could have done a better survey than Ed did. He'd come down to the boat, sit at the settee, drink a cup of coffee, ask a few questions without ever looking at a thing, and then charge us a couple of hundred bucks. It would have been more productive to take two one-hundred-dollar bills and run them through a shredder than it was to have Ed survey the boat. But we were stuck with him since the only other surveyor was even worse. At least, I liked Ed, even if his surveys left a lot to be desired.

This weird story twist caused my laughter. In the early '90s I was working for Ketchikan Public Utilities (KPU) as a powerhouse mechanic. One day I was sitting in the lunch room, drinking a cup of coffee before work started, when Ed walked in the door followed by a man named Gary. KPU regularly hired temporary laborers to work in the maintenance department, but usually they were college-aged kids –– not two middle-aged guys. These laborers would help us with everything from cleaning in the powerhouses to cutting brush along the penstocks that feed water to the hydro powerhouses. Anyway, when Ed and Gary started, we were rebuilding one of the large diesel engines in the Bailey Powerhouse. The engine we were rebuilding was a V-18 with cylinders so large a person can crawl inside them. The rods were over five feet long; the injectors were a foot long and weighed about forty pounds each. Huge, or even gargantuan, might be better terms to describe that engine than large.

When working on a diesel engine that is that big, mechanics use a lot of rags –– so many rags that we kept a large industrial-grade washing machine going full time washing the oil, diesel, and grease out of the rags. Since the boss had told me to put Ed and Gary to work helping us, I assigned them to wash the rags between helping us tear the machine apart, clean and sort parts. I told them where they'd find two 55-gallon drums full of rags, and to put them in the washer that was in the locker room. I continued, saying, "You'll find a cardboard barrel of laundry soap right across from the washing machine. Depending on how dirty the rags are, put a ½ to ¾ of a cup of soap in the machine. When the washer is done, put the rags in the dryer and when they are dry, put the clean rags in the clean rag barrels." I thought these instructions were clear and simple –– wrong.

The diesel engine we were working on was located on the second floor of the powerhouse, and the locker room where the washing machine was located was on the ground floor. At one point I headed down the stairs and was a little surprised to see soap suds coming out of one of the floor drains. But when I looked towards the locker room, about 75 feet away, my jaw dropped to the floor. There was a four-foot-high wall of soap bubbles oozing from the door to the locker room like a slow-moving flow of bubbly lava. In the locker room I saw bubbles coming out of the top and back of the washing machine, and out the drain of the mop sink. Past the row of lockers on the left and right, the mop sink, washer and dryer all the way to the back wall were bubbles growing out of the shower drain nearly to the ceiling. When I saw the 18-inch diameter wall fan blowing bubbles out of the back wall, I laughed. Now I'm going to show my age; Ed and Gary had made an oversized Lawrence Welk bubble machine that was blasting bubbles out of the powerplant. What was extra amusing to me -- there was no turning off the bubble-maker until the large front-loading washing machine ran its full cycle and its door could be unlocked.

For the next hour or so Ed and Gary shoveled and swept soap suds out the front door of the powerhouse, and then they had one heck of a mess to clean. There is a high possibility that the locker room hadn't been that clean since it was brand new. One of them poured in ¾ of a gallon of liquid soap they found under the mop sink we used for mopping the floor instead of the ½ to a ¾ cup of laundry soap I told them to use.

Their next screw-up was courtesy of Ed. We had finished rebuilding the engine, and I was now working at one of the hydro plants. Before I left the Bailey power plant, I was to show them, who by now had earned the nicknames Frank and Ernest after the cartoon caricatures, where the floor paint was so they could paint the floors in two storage rooms. Right at 8:00 am I walked them to the paint locker and showed them the epoxy boat deck paint we used on all the powerhouse floors. Since Ed was a marine surveyor, I figured he would know about marine paints -- wrong again. After showing them the two rooms that needed to be painted, I said they should be extra careful to read the instructions on the can, offered them the Material Safety Data Sheets (MSDS) paperwork on the hazards of using a toxic paint like that brand of epoxy, recommended they wear protective clothing, ventilated the area, and asked them to wear respirators if they felt the air was not good enough with ventilation. Lastly, I said to be sure and mix the paint as per the directions and be sure to mix it well.

When I returned to Bailey at the end of the day, I was delighted to stick my head in the two rooms and thought things looked good. However, the next morning when I arrived to work before everyone else, the paint was still wet. When Ed arrived, I asked him if they had mixed the paint well and he assured me they did. I figured it was just taking longer to cure than usual and I headed back out to the hydro plant. That afternoon back at the Bailey Powerhouse, Ed confessed his mistake. It ends up he was concerned, so he called the toll-free technical support number that was on the can. When he asked why the paint was taking so long to cure the customer service rep asked him, "Did you mix the two parts equally?" To which Ed confessed his reply, "Two parts?" They didn't add the catalyst to the paint, so it was never going to cure. Ugh, now how we were going to fix that?

The next morning, I called the toll-free number. I was told we might have to use a special solvent to remove the paint, but we could try to mix the paint properly, repaint the floor and if we're lucky, the uncatalyzed paint might cure. I'm happy to report that it did cure, but what a mess it was to repaint a floor that had wet paint on it? Fortunately, that fell to Ed and Gary, or should I say, Frank and Ernest?

During the six months Ed and Gary worked for us, I had to watch them like a hawk. Even then, they continued to make all of us laugh with their antics, and there was no doubt that their nicknames fit. They somehow had a knack of turning a simple job into an epic misadventure.

When Connie and I moved to Sitka, it was again time to have our beloved sailboat, Terra Nova, surveyed. We called Stef, and this time we had a real survey done by a real professional. Stef looked under every floorboard, inspected the engine, made sure the batteries were all topped off, made sure the bilge pump worked and even made sure the anchor windless was in working order. Ed never did any of the things I just mentioned. Just like Ed obviously didn't read the instructions on the floor paint, he always did a half-assed job when it came to surveying our boat. In contrast, Stef did a professional job and even found a problem with the installation on our oil-fired heating stove, which had been overlooked by Ed several times. I say overlooked, but in reality, Ed never looked and likely wouldn't have known better anyway.

When I recall the time I worked at KPU, I can't help but wonder if that work could be responsible for my ALS? I was much too lackadaisical when it came to taking precautions working with chemicals and welding fumes. Often, I was totally covered in diesel fuel, or partially covered in oil, cleaning solvents, industrial paints, or breathing welding fumes that were as thick as a London fog. All that exposure surely wasn't good for me, and I now harp on my grandsons about taking precautions when working around those things. I'll never know what caused my ALS, but that doesn't mean that I'll give up on being curious. Nor will I give up on living life the best that I can under the circumstances. So, even if I feel totally awkward not being able to talk when I attend an event like we did yesterday, I'll still enjoy it. One of the things I love is classical music, and fulfilling that love is one of the things that makes life worth living.

Hatred and Intolerance

7 May 2019

Is it just me or does it seem like there is less tolerance and more hatred in our country today than there was in years past? Maybe it's social media that highlights the hate that has always been there? Or, could social media be the fertilizer that makes that hate and intolerance grow? I don't know the answer, but it saddens me.

I hate ALS and everything it's doing to me and other ALS sufferers. However, I'm also grateful that ALS has helped teach me to be more tolerant of others. In the past five years, I've been blessed to be exposed to all types of healthcare people with all tones of skin color. I would have to be blind in more ways than one not to see the good in healthcare workers that are different than I am. The same can be said about anyone who has spent time in a big city hospital. How can some of those same people spread the hatred they do in their Facebook posts?

I've long ago lost track of how many times I've checked in at the front desk of the three major hospitals in Seattle. In addition to people who look like me, I've been checked in by an amicable transgender person, an equally friendly gay man, an always smiling and helpful woman confined to a wheelchair, and a whole host of other helpful people. I've had blood drawn by phlebotomists of several different nationalities, including a couple that appear to have an English vocabulary of fewer than a hundred words. Other than my local doctor's office phlebotomist, my favorite is a Vietnamese man of about my age that I assume is likely a refugee from the Vietnam War. I'll talk about the myriad of nurses I've seen in a minute, but first I'm going to talk about the doctors.

It would be hard for me to put an exact number of how many doctors I've seen in the last five years, but certainly over a hundred. There have been women and men doctors of all skin colors and ethnicities. There have been several doctors who are new to America, including my latest neurologist, a woman from China. I owe my life to a few of those doctors.

In the summer of 2015, after a year of doctors trying to figure out what was wrong with me, it was discovered that I had a tumor on my pituitary gland that would require surgery to remove. After a couple of months of drug therapy to prepare me for the operation, a date was set for early October. Since the pituitary gland sits at the base of the brain and between the two carotid arteries and near the optic nerve, removing the tumor is very tricky and requires a very skilled surgeon. In my case, that surgeon was an immigrant and, judging by his name and accent, from Iran. And, by the last name of my anesthesiologist for that surgery, I assumed he was Jewish. I, of course, was asleep during the six-and-a-half-hour operation, but what I do remember was when I was wheeled into the operating room, first, was how big it was, and second, how many people were in the room preparing for the surgery. There were at least a dozen people, and even under the surgical masks, I could see several different ethnic backgrounds. I was welcomed to the surgery suite by an African American man built like a Seattle Seahawks linebacker. He said he was the head surgical nurse and assured me that everyone in the room was there to make sure I had an excellent outcome.

Marcel LaPerriere

During the close-to-a-month I was in the hospital or staying in the attached hotel, my room was cleaned daily by a couple of friendly Muslim women wearing hijabs, and my meals were often served by Hispanic or Filipino people. I often saw a man pushing a cart by my hospital room, and by the head turban he wore, I assumed he was Sikh. And when I had an adverse reaction to penicillin that nearly killed me, a very compassionate Hispanic doctor treated me.

Now let's talk about nurses, many of whom deserve sainthood. In the week I stayed in intensive care, and then another week in a regular room, I was taken care of by both women and men nurses of Hispanic, African American, Caucasian, Filipino, Indian, and Asian descent, and even by a very polite male nurse from Vietnam. A couple of nurses stand out as extra caring: first, there was the nurse from Vietnam that I've already mentioned. Every time he'd come into the room he'd bow and ask how he could be of service. Then there was the young African American night nurse, who always took an extra step of being apologetic when she'd have to wake me to give me a shot. She was even kind when she had to work two back-to-back days of a fifteen-hour shift because they were shorthanded.

In grade school we were taught that America is the melting pot of the world, making us a great nation of immigrants. We were also taught the first-Amendment, including this part, *"Congress shall make no law respecting an establishment of religion."* With those words enshrined in our Constitution, how can so many be so intolerant of those who don't worship the same God they do? There are some bad Muslim people, just like there are bad Christian people or those of any other religion. And in recent news there are even some bad Buddhists. But that doesn't mean all people from any of those religions are bad. We need to solve our illegal immigration issues, but, just because we have a problem, it doesn't make all Hispanic people bad people. The Bible says, *"He that is without sin among you, let him cast the first stone...?"* With that, how can we forget that our European ancestors intentionally or unintentionally did their best to annihilate the indigenous people of the Americas?

It scares me when I see such hatred in posts on Facebook. Sadly, they give me a better understanding of how something as horrific as the Holocaust happened. Sadder still, a large percentage of Americans don't know about the Holocaust or deny it ever happened. As a person who has visited the Dachau concentration camp, where all these years later you can still smell death, I can assure you that it did happen.

It sucks to have ALS; however, it has given me a chance to see the value in people, women and men, big and tall, small and short, black, brown, white, gay, transgender or any other label you want to put on them. Inherently, most people are good. And when a person is not good, we need to deal with that one person on an individual basis, not label everyone that falls in their category as bad. As a person who leans towards the progressive side, politically, online I have been called all sorts of ugly names. I let those names roll off my back while feeling sorry for the person who is filled with enough hate to call me those names. I just hope that these folks someday will realize that hate, like all negative things, only sparks more hatred and intolerance of others, including themselves. What's wrong with giving people the benefit of the doubt until they prove otherwise? If your religion or political beliefs compel you to hate others, you need to look for another religion or change your political views. Hate begets hate. Intolerance begets more intolerance.

Socks

10 May 2019

It's hard to believe I could get up in the morning, dress and be out of the house on my way to work in under ten minutes. Nowadays it can take five to ten minutes just to put on my socks.

Bathing and dressing ourselves gives those of us living with ALS a little independence. I'm lucky that I can still do both, now over five years into this journey. Things I used to think were simple are now not only more time consuming but take more energy than I would have ever thought possible. Take socks –– UGH! They are hard to put on and even harder to take off. I find that sock-aids are of little use putting socks on, and are no help at all taking them off.

Here again is where I'm lucky. I married a super-talented wife who likes to sew. She came up with a sock solution that she now makes for me. After three prototypes, we figured out that a zipper-up-the-front sock [see photo] works best for me. Velcro on the front and inside of the socks didn't do the job for me.

Fortunately, my wife is an expert on sewing and designing anything with cloth. She used a pair of my regular socks to make a pattern, cut out the pieces from a soft flannel cloth and sewed them together into a custom sock. I tried each design a few times, until I decided the front zipper worked best. The zipper is a heavy-duty zipper like you find on a backpack, with a good zipper pull. These socks are much easier to put on, and taking them off is a breeze. Taking off socks was harder than putting them on. By the time I'd get them off, I'd be spent, and it was a good thing I was heading directly to bed.

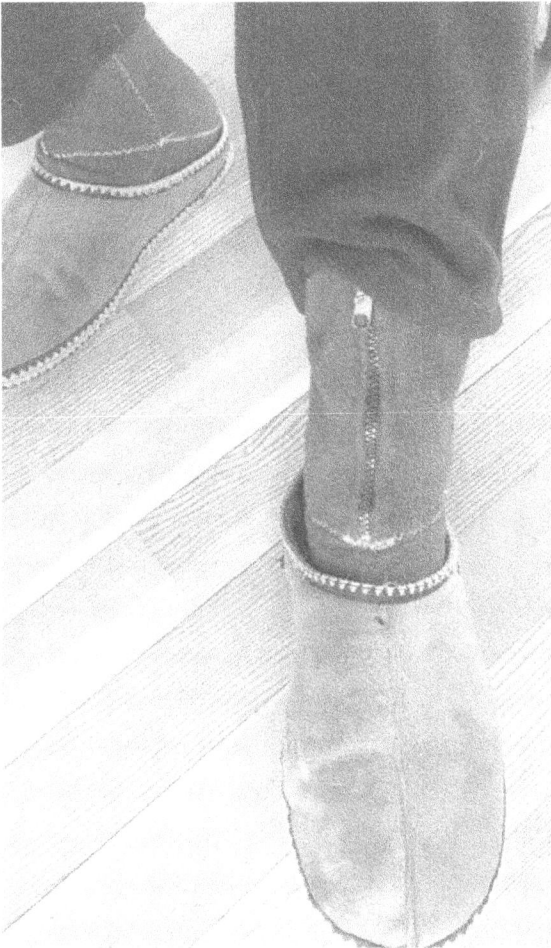

May 2019. Along with easy-on socks, I almost always wear open-heal slippers or clog-type shoes.

Being married to a seamstress has even more advantages. Connie made me soft cloth armrests for my manual wheelchair after I started getting pressure sores on my arms, and a special pillow that I use under my ankles to prevent getting pressure sores on my heals. And, she even made fitted satin sheets for my hospital type bed after we couldn't find any to buy. The satin not only helps me roll over at night, but the softer cloth keeps me from getting bed sores.

As I write this, we are celebrating 47 years together. We have never been into giving each other gifts on our birthdays, Christmas or our anniversary. However, I know what a wonderful gift she has given me with these easy on and off socks. Yep, I'm one lucky guy.

Trilogy 100

15 May 2019

On Monday of this week I began a forced education into a subject that I'd just as soon not be learning about –– how to use the Trilogy 100, a noninvasive ventilator. That said, I'm grateful that we have the technology that will make breathing easier for me and could literally extend my life.

The journey to get the Trilogy ventilator was like many other medical issues we've dealt with. By the fall of 2018 it was becoming more and more evident that I'd need mechanical help breathing. We started with Dr. Kirtland, the last pulmonologist I saw. He must have agreed, because he quickly wrote a prescription for the Trilogy. But Medicare rejected the order because it had been more than six months since I had last seen him. That's when we learned that we could have asked Dr. Hunter, my primary care physician, to write the prescription. But we were again rejected, this time because I was still using a bilevel positive airway pressure (BIPAP) machine. Medicare was paying for the BIPAP with a thirteen-month rent-to-own contract, and there was still a bit over two months left on the contract when we learned that it would disqualify payment for the Trilogy. Medicare did give us the option of giving up the BI-PAP, but I didn't want to do that because it would be hard for me to transfer the Trilogy from the living room to my bedroom by myself. If I can't transfer by myself, I would be dependent on Connie to always be here when I want to take a nap –– something neither of us wanted. Also, the way they made it sound, I'd have to ship the BIPAP back before the Trilogy could be sent, and I can't sleep without the aid of a machine to help me breathe. So we waited until the BIPAP's thirteen-month contract had finished and almost a month more before the Trilogy could be shipped from Anchorage to our home in Sitka.

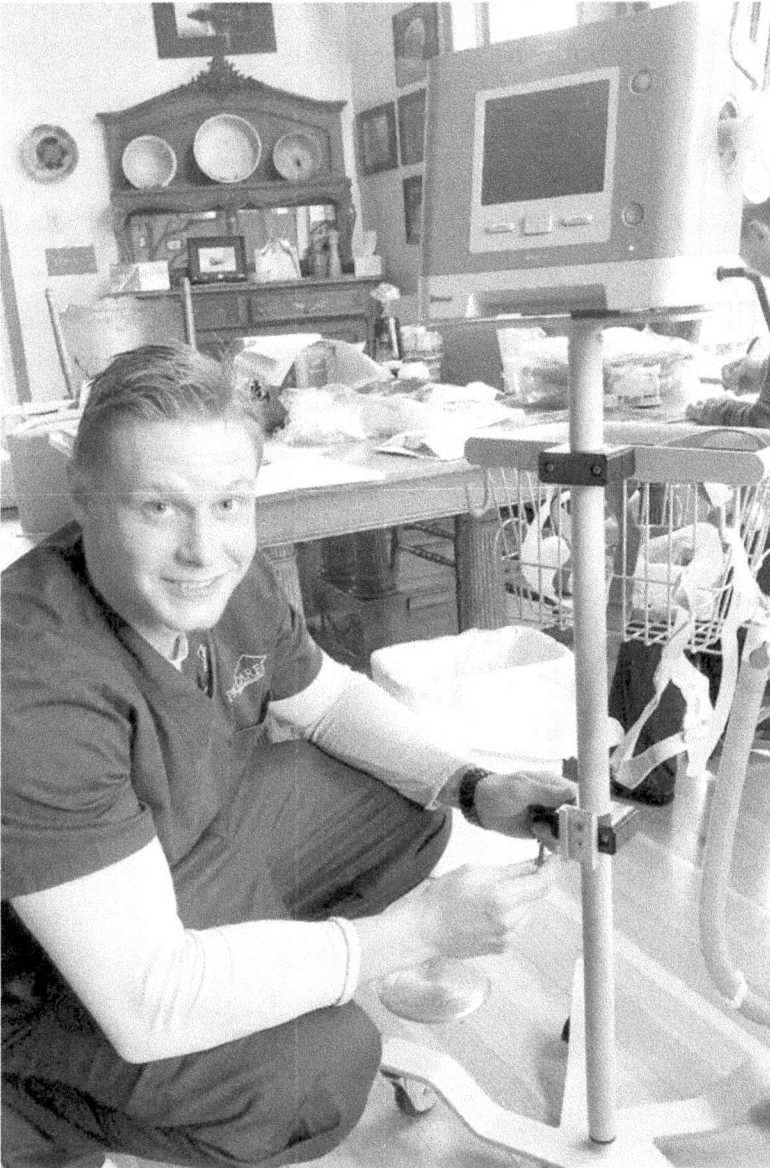

May 2019. Austin Sycks from PROCARE adjusts a bracket on the Trilogy stand.

Getting the hands-on training Medicare required for the Trilogy worried me. I thought that it might delay the delivery of the Trilogy again. I figured we'd have to travel to either Anchorage or Seattle, and travel by air is getting hard. That would mean we'd have to wait until we could catch the ferry for an extended trip. Imagine my surprise when we were told that the Trilogy, along with a person to do the training, would be sent to Sitka to set up and educate us on how to use it.

As a person who is always early, I appreciated it when Austin Sycks, the Respiratory Tec from PROCARE, showed up about ten minutes early. He walked Connie and me through all the steps to the machine, and because we are not in a major city where in-person support is easy, he showed us many adjustments most patients would not do. After more than an hour and a half of training, I understand why Medicare wants the user and caregiver to have quite detailed use and trouble-shooting instructions. Even though I would just as soon not need the Trilogy, I'm still grateful for both the device and the training we received. I'll be even more thankful if the Trilogy gives me more energy and a longer life. Time will tell.

Fall

16 May 2019

I fell today for the first time in months. I wasn't hurt, but I couldn't get off the floor without help. Even I was surprised at how weak I've gotten.

This morning I was being lazy. I kept nodding back off to sleep, but I still got up before Connie, which has been the usual thing for us throughout our married life. Even though I now need around eleven hours of sleep in a day, I still can't break the habit of getting up early. When I got up at 6:30, I was already feeling a little guilty for sleeping in.

After getting up, I made my way to the bathroom using my walker, which has been the custom for nearly the last two years. After using the toilet, I again used my walker to make all of the three-foot walk to the sink. I washed my hands and my face while holding onto the vanity and sink, and when I turned to grab the walker, bam, my left knee just buckled. I knew I was going down, so I just let myself fall, and I did my best to keep my head from hitting the wall, toilet or floor. I also discovered I must have some sort of unique falling talent, because even though it was my left knee that failed me, I somehow ended up on my right side. During the fall, I kicked the walker across the room which hit the wall, making a small divot in the sheetrock and a fair bit of noise.

Marcel LaPerriere

That racket was followed a split-second later by Connie yelling, "Oh no." In less time than it took me to type, "Oh no," Connie was standing over me. She knew I wasn't hurt, because I was laughing when she arrived. As many times as both Connie and I have cheated death by falling while we were doing extreme sports like climbing or caving, I had to laugh at the irony of falling in my own bathroom. The next few minutes went by with me going between laughter and crying, because it was becoming apparent I wasn't going to be getting off the floor anytime soon. We both kept trying, and somehow in confusion, Connie tripped on the walker, which made both of us laugh, but sadly she somehow cut her leg in the process.

Since we have in-floor radiant heat, most mornings when I get up the tile floor is toasty warm, but as luck would have it, today the heat wasn't on, and the floor was ice cold. So with Connie's help, and ten minutes or so of slithering, I was back on the much warmer wooden bedroom floor. There I hoped I could grab onto the bed legs, roll onto my belly and then, with help, get up on my knees. I did succeed in rolling onto my stomach, but the PEG feeding tube made that too uncomfortable as it pushed into my gut. By this time, Connie had called the fire department's non-emergency number.

Connie put a blanket on me, and in less than five minutes, a large fireman showed up. Because we live in a small town and we know the Fire Chief and many of the employees and volunteers that work at the Fire Department, I was a little surprised that I'd never seen this man before. However, like most firemen, he knew what to do. Pulling my arms, he lifted me into a sitting position, and then got behind me, grabbed me under the arms, and lifted me part way up while Connie rolled the wheelchair under me.

As is often the case with bulbar ALS, I was overcome with emotions and once again went from crying to laughing all in a minute or two. As I cried, I realized how grateful I am that we have such an excellent fire department so close to us. Even with the fire department as close as it is, and even though he called, "Call us anytime," as he walked out the door, we now know we need to get a lift.

As Connie and I talked about getting the lift, I typed into my phone and hit Talk, "Now all you're going to need to do is learn how to tie a hangman's noose." I have to laugh at what I know is coming down the line, or surely, I'll cry.

Marcel LaPerriere

Lump-Pa

19 May 2019

When my grandson Nate, who is now 13, and his older brother, Blake, who is now 17, were little, they would sometimes jokingly call me Grump-Pa. I'd play along by pretending to be extra grumpy. Nowadays, a better name for me would be Lump-Pa. I say that because I often feel as if I'm an extra-large lump of worthless detritus. I feel I have little value to my family or anyone anymore. I can't help with the household chores, and, other than my pension and Social Security, can't contribute to the family income. I'm a drain on the family and on society –– at least that's how I often feel.

Since Blake was born, followed by Nate, and then Dane, who is now 9, the boys have come to our house most Sundays. Today we decided to go to the park where we often walk Bella and, while there, look at a newly built eagle nest. Blake even grabbed a pair of binoculars so we could get a better look at the nest. When we got to the park, Dane ran ahead as he always does, followed by Nate. When I caught up to them, I zipped ahead, because the nest is well hidden, and I didn't want them to run too far. I stopped at the best place to see the nest. Blake soon caught up, took a quick look, handed the binoculars to Nate, and then ran off to look at the base of the tree that the nest is in. Connie,

Dane, and Bella passed us, showing little interest in looking at the nest. After a quick glance with the binoculars, Nate started to run off, until I beeped my horn to get his attention. I, too, wanted to look, and I did for a few seconds while Nate was jumping around showing no patience to stand there holding the binocular covers. Just then some tourists walked by, and I pointed up and pointed to Nate hoping he'd tell the tourist about the nest. He didn't, and I didn't have time to pull out my phone before they were gone. Nate then ran ahead, and while he ran off the trail to also look at the base of the tree, I typed in my phone, "What I was trying to tell you was you should have pointed out the eagle's nest to those people; it would have made their day." When I showed Nate what I had written, he nodded his head then and ran ahead.

Besides walking Bella, I had thought the reason we went to the park was to spend some time looking at the eagle nest, so I was a little frustrated that no one wanted to spend any time doing that. I was also frustrated that I couldn't communicate my feelings. So I sped up to catch them as they waited further up the trail. When I approached them, I saw that Bella had a stick stuck in her mouth and was pawing at it. Everyone was totally oblivious to Bella's plight, and my frustration continued to build as I kept grunting and pointing at a dog who was in distress. Dane and Nate ran ahead again, which meant that Bella started chasing them. I was worried about Bella, so I beeped my horn. Connie stopped, which made Bella stop, and to my relief, I saw Bella had somehow gotten the stick out of her mouth.

My frustration continued to build all the rest of the way back to the van. On two occasions, tourists blocked my path forward, and since everyone was far ahead of me, they could not help me ask people to move. The frustration was nearing a boiling point when a woman stood totally blocking the trail to take a photo of a fern. Ugh. It's times like that when not being able to talk is overwhelming, and that frustration sparks my anger. I didn't mind waiting for the lady, but I would have appreciated a little help from my family communicating, especially since I was already feeling pressured to hurry. After the woman moved, I once again caught up, and we made it back to the van and headed home.

As Connie backed in the garage, she asked the boys to give her a hand carrying some dirt out of the back of the truck and down the hill to our front yard. When the van was parked, she asked them to give me room so that I could get out of the van. They started playing a game with some old boxes at the bottom of the ramp which blocked my exit –– not a big deal, except I wanted to get inside to use the restroom. After a couple of minutes, they moved and ran off with me following them. Again, not a big deal, but no one stayed to hold open the gate on our walkway that keeps Bella from running out in the road. Small, because I can easily open it on my own, but it demonstrated that, yes, I'm just a big lump of detritus, with no value.

I got into the house okay, and as I stood up to take off my coats before I transferred to my manual chair, Bella scratched at the door in desperation to get out. I have no idea why they let her in the house, since every one of them knows that Bella is going to want to be part of the action. Since taking off my coat is no easy task, and it would take a few minutes to transfer to my manual chair, I sat back down in my power chair and powered over to the door to let Bella outside. By this time, my anger and frustration had built to a point that I was having what I can best describe as a feeling like a panic attack. That feeling then manifested itself into the fight or flight mode. Since I can't fight, I followed Bella outside, made sure she was not near the gate, and I rolled back out to the street, totally forgetting that I had to pee, as I started my flight. The sensation of having to pee was no longer critical, but escape was.

Where we live, the sidewalk is only on one side of the street, opposite our house. I tilted my chair back to prevent the foot rest from hitting the curb and, with a quick glance trying to see around the curve in the road, I zipped across the street, not totally caring if a speeding car came a little too fast around the corner. Feeling like a lump of crap, why should I care? I headed down the street to the duck park on the lake, thinking, "If I motor my wheelchair out onto the dock, stand up and fall forward into the lake, this nightmare of living with ALS would all be over in a minute or two." I'm happy to say by the time I had reached the park, I had come to my senses. I turned my chair around, and as a light rain fell on my face, I headed back home. I was reasonably sure no one would even know I'd been gone. As I entered the gate, I heard the boys and Connie talking in the yard, and I rolled into the house undetected. The urge to pee came back, and I started the process of taking my coats off, transferred into my manual chair, and rolled into the restroom. After peeing and washing my hands, I headed back out into the living room, just as everyone was coming inside. As I suspected, no one knew I had been gone ten minutes.

I try hard not to throw myself a pity party, but the frustration of not being able to talk, then the irrational anger, coupled with my empathy for a little dog that I loved, a little dog that everyone seemed to be ignoring, made the pity party inevitable. This pity party made me better understand and empathize with other people living with ALS that post things on Facebook about depression, anger, and loneliness. I also better understood why a woman who is the caregiver to her husband recently posted that she thinks her husband hates her. I don't think he hates her, but he hasn't learned how to deal with his own battles dealing with their ALS Monster.

Just when I think the ALS Monster can't win against me, I have a day like today. The Monster won today's battle, as it will eventually win the war. I can't give the Monster the satisfaction of letting it win day-to-day battles. I need to be more patient, accept that boys will be kids, and that means I must learn to be more tolerant.

Postscript, 21 May 2019: After Connie read the essay above, we talked, and I must admit, I wasn't being fair to her. It's not easy for her to worry about me, take care of a high-maintenance dog, and manage three high energy boys. She once again assured me that I shouldn't feel worthless, and after a couple of days reflecting on one lousy day, I still have value. I'm still a husband, a father, and a grandfather. I might not be able to do the things I used to, but I can still contribute not only to my family, but to society. I write these essays hoping to help others deal with their own battles. I also continue to volunteer work. Just yesterday, I spent much of the day assessing and then writing a paper with my suggestions on how to do some restoration work on a historic building. And I've recently started a Facebook page called Tips for Handicap Accessibility Modifications. I'll keep on contributing what and when I can, even as the ALS Monster continues to take abilities from me.

Hope

31 May 2019

In most cases when someone finds out they might, or do, have ALS, they are overcome with a feeling of dread, and there is a loss of hope. With the statics of a life expectancy of two to five years, who can blame them? But dread is like cancer and builds on itself. To fight that dread, and other negativity, "Hope" can go a long way toward making life worth living, even if it means you or a loved one is living with ALS.

As I was wrapping up this book, my ALS Facebook friend, Hossein, shared a poignant post that captured what it is like to have ALS" or witness someone who does. With the help of Hossein, I tracked down the author of the post, Al Rogers, who gave me permission to quote his touching words that follow:

> *How can someone without ALS understand the total vulnerability and helplessness of not being able to raise a hand to feed yourself or drink. Of not being able to clean oneself after a bowel movement, put on a pair of socks, or pick up a phone to text, or use a pen. Not being able to lift your arm back up when it slips off the bed or roll over. Then not daring to go out in public because public lavatories are not suited for the needs of an ALS patient, or when eating in a restaurant is no longer possible because having to be*

fed, or swallowing is no longer possible without drooling, or not possible at all. That even scratching one's nose is no longer possible. The idea that speech will no longer be possible without technology that one may or not be able to afford and even then, may eventually be no longer an option.

Advocacy for ALS is well-intentioned. There have been advocates who have ALS who have made powerful arguments and valiant efforts in this regard, However most advocates who do not have ALS or the strong direct connection to this disease have the handicap of this reality being blurred in the abstract and having the option of being able to disconnect from the direness of the ALS reality. Even the scientists involved in research fall in this category who are either on the periphery of ALS research or accidentally drawn in by other non-related research.

Only a small 5% to 10% of ALS cases that are genetically linked have brought some glimmer of possible progress. The rest of the ALS cases are still an enigma. Most of the medical treatments or drugs only dubiously extend life by a month or two with much confusion of when to take a drug like Riluzole or whether the expensive process of taking Radicava is worth it. For pharmaceutical companies, the motivation is clear, but for the patient, it's a matter of desperation.

The ALS patient knows that he or she is going to die. The issues are how to deal with the daily struggles of living to be able to find reasons for living! To be able to find something to enjoy in life and things to share with loved ones without simply feeling a burden to those loved ones. To be able to feel that someone understands.

This is why support groups are so important. For patients to be able to share their experiences and struggles gives more comfort than one might realize. It's not sympathy but mutual understanding. It is a confounding dilemma for an ALS patient to hear from perhaps good intentioned friends or others who say things like, "Oh. I hope you feel better."

Then the frustration of dealing with the many healthcare professionals that have little or no experience with, nor knowledge of ALS. The misdiagnoses that can drag on for as much as two years before the realization that ALS is the cause of symptoms. The reactions of insurance companies that claim certain services or technologies aren't necessary.

I bring this up because while ALS patients are all too aware in every fiber of their being of these things, those of us who are on the periphery need to be reminded. The fight needs to go on.

The realization that ALS is one of the ghastliest incomprehensible & tragic diseases of mankind has to be brought home to the government, insurance companies, and the scientific/medical world. But also, so important is to help society understand the reality of the helpless world of the ALS!

During the process of getting permission to use Al's words, I learned that he lost his wife, Cheryl to ALS in 2017. I was once again touched when he wrote this in an email to me.

"I was faced with how to go on without my wife. I realized that I still had so much love for her and instead of perpetual mourning, I realized that I wanted to extend that love to the ALS community. I started the closed group page and became active with the New Mexico chapter of ALS Association."

I have since joined a closed ALS support group. Who better to understand the challenges dealt the ALS card than Al, who lived a life of a spouse and caregiver to a person with ALS?

I have titled the ending essay, "Hope," for several reasons. Because people have ALS doesn't mean that they or their loved ones can't have hope. Al's continued active support is also part of that hope. The old saying that there is strength in numbers applies to hope, too. A support group not only helps me feel hope, but it makes me happy when I can help or give hope to others. When Connie and I joined in one support group's conference, we gained hope when one participant said he'd been living with ALS for sixteen years. That gave me hope that I might get to see my three grandsons grow into adults with their own families.

In just the last few months there is good news from Australia about a drug called CuATSM. It shows promise for slowing the disease, and that gives us hope. Even some over the counter supplements like CBD oil or L-Serine are showing promise, which gives us hope as well. We all hope for happiness, even when living with ALS. We hope for the love of a family. We hope that new drugs or therapies will be discovered. We hope that we are not pitied. And, for sure we hope for a cure. Mostly, I hope this book has been helpful to you. *The Adventure Continues*, and I hope to be around for many more years.

Acknowledgements

I owe Dana Anderson a big thank you once again for her professional work compiling my essays and putting them into this book. She did such a great job with my first book, *Just Another Adventure: Living with Amyotrophic Lateral Sclerosis*, that I was thrilled when she said she'd do this book as well. August 11, 2019

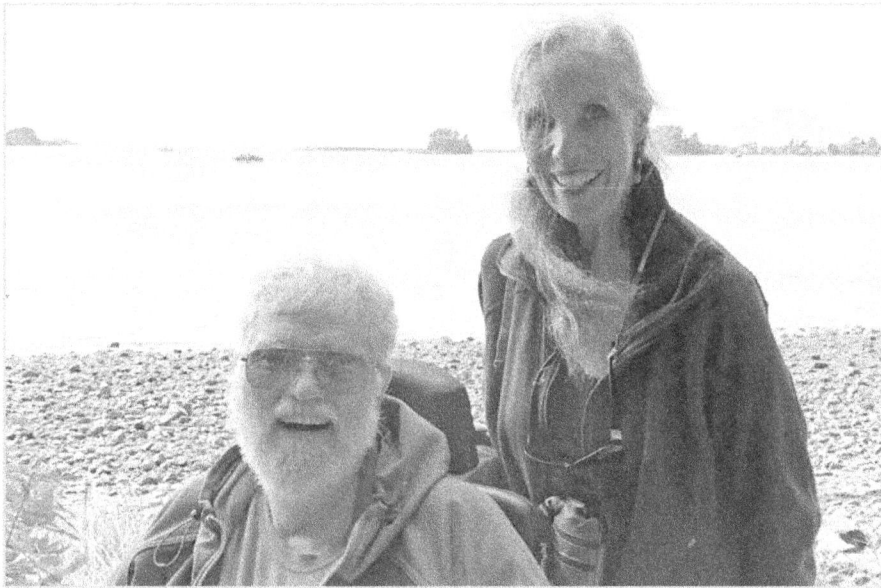

Dana traveled from Anchorage to Sitka, Alaska to hand-deliver the latest manuscript draft to me. After a yummy taco-pizza lunch with Connie and our three grandsons, Dana, Connie, and Dane joined me on a stroll and roll in Sitka National Historic Park, where this photo was taken.

Thanks also to Max and Bonnie Cottrell for their help editing many of the essays, Margot Demarais, and to my son Zach and his wife Jenn Lawlor for their help editing essays in this book and my first book.

Of course, the biggest thank you needs to go to my wife, Connie, who is always the first to read my writing, the first to make suggestions, and correct my endless mistakes.

Thank you all. I couldn't have done it without your help.

Marcel LaPerriere

About the Author

Like many Alaskans, Marcel was employed in a multitude of jobs including machinist, powerhouse mechanic, climbing and fitness gym owner, web hosting service owner, online retail store owner that sold Alaska-made arts and crafts, logger and sawmill operator, carpenter, director of maintenance at a small liberal arts college, and building contractor. He even did a year-long stint as a recruiter, traveling the state of Alaska looking for candidates for placement in a maritime academy. Not one to shy away from a challenge, Marcel thrived on hard work and hard play. He was an active scuba diver, logging over a thousand dives, a mountain climber and a caver. With his wife, Connie, he helped discover, explore and map many caves in Southeast Alaska.

As ALS started to creep into Marcel's life, he elected to look at the disease as just another adventure; one that had been forced on him. He and Connie decided early on to do all they could to fight ALS, but they accepted that a diagnosis of ALS, at this time, is always a death sentence. They make the most of each day, and live life happy in their acceptance of the horrific disease that ALS is. As Marcel lost his ability to speak, he started writing. This book and his first book, *Just Another Adventure: Living with Amyotrophic Lateral Scleroses* are the results of that writing. Marcel is currently working on a book of personal stories from his life, *The Path to Adventure*, and, with any luck, one more book about living with ALS.

The Adventure Continues

Marcel LaPerriere

The Adventure Continues

Marcel LaPerriere

www.ingramcontent.com/pod-product-compliance
Lightning Source LLC
Chambersburg PA
CBHW080358030426
42334CB00024B/2912

9 780578 524887